COASTAL YACHT
NAVIGATION

COASTAL YACHT NAVIGATION

Craig Coutts

REED

By the same author:
Blue Water Yacht Navigation
Boat Navigation for Beginners

Published by Reed Books, a division of Reed Publishing
(NZ) Ltd, 39 Rawene Road, Birkenhead, Auckland.
Associated companies, branches and representatives
throughout the world.

ISBN 0 7900 0112 8

© 1988, 1993 Craig Coutts

First published 1981
Revised edition 1988, 1989, 1991
New edition 1993
Reprinted 1995, 1997

Typeset by Glenfield Graphics Ltd
and Typocrafters Ltd, Auckland

Printed in Singapore

Front cover photograph courtesy of *Boating World*.
Back cover photograph courtesy of Bill Barry,
Boating New Zealand

Contents

Acknowledgements

I would like to thank the following for permission to reproduce material in this book: The Hydrographer, Royal New Zealand Navy, for portions of charts NZ 532 and 5322 and extracts from NZ 201; the Director Hydrographic Operations, Royal Australian Navy, for the Australian Notices to Mariners; GP Publications Ltd for use of the range table and the secondary ports table extracts from the *New Zealand Nautical Almanac*, 1990/91 edition; the Director, New Zealand Meteorological Service, for cloud types and weather satellite photographs; Bi-rola Rule Ltd for the chart protractor; Trans Pacific Marine Ltd and A. Foster & Co. Ltd for photographs of a steering compass, grid steering compass, prism sight, parallel rulers and navigation instruments.

Introduction

Navigation is a very practical subject. *Coastal Yacht Navigation* is a concise book for the beginner, stripped to its practical essentials, designed for use by yacht, motor yacht and power boat owners. The aim is to give the reader the essential information to conduct a craft with safety in harbour or on coastal passages. I have taken care to point out any pitfalls in the various procedures and to give practical advice which may differ from the theoretical or textbook solutions. While intended to help the novice develop his skills offshore, the book also contains hints for the more experienced reader and explains some simple procedures neglected elsewhere.

The book is not intended to be read at a single sitting; indeed, it should prove a useful reference work long after the reader has gained a working knowledge of the subject. In my experience, the competent navigator is not the person who thinks he knows it all, but the one who realises that there is always a little more to learn. No two sets of circumstances are ever exactly the same and the best course of action must be decided in the light of a person's knowledge and experience. Where the competent navigator scores is in knowing the best book to refer to for advice on tackling the type of situation in which he finds himself at a given time. Then, having refreshed his memory, he can adapt the information to solving the particular problem on hand. This usually takes a little commonsense, not a degree in higher mathematics.

There have been some small but significant changes since this book was last revised and these are reflected in the diagrams and text. The use of more recent aids to coastal navigation such as radar is included, as is a section on meteorology for information and for future reference.

However, *Coastal Yacht Navigation* can take you just so far. With the basics under your belt, the only way to become a good practical navigator is to go to sea and put the book learning into practice. My advice is to get out there and go to it.

Craig Coutts
Auckland, 1993

1

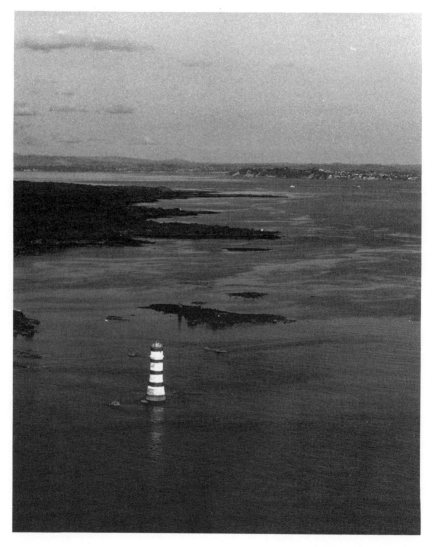

Fig. 1 *Lighthouse*   *Courtesy Auckland Coast Guard*

Chapter One
Basics

What's the good of Mercator's North Poles and Equators, Tropics, Zones, and Meridian Lines?
          Lewis Carroll, The Hunting of the Snark

The above quotation asks a reasonable question, but who was this fellow Mercator anyway? The answers will be found in this and later chapters, together with explanations of other terms used in coastal navigation.

Navigation in general is the art of taking a boat from one place to another in safety as economically as possible. With the price of oil these days, only an idiot would waste the stuff by taking the long way round.

Coastal navigation in particular concerns that part of a sea passage in which the navigator has the land on one side of the boat and the open sea on the other. Channel navigation is concerned with conducting a craft through narrow channels with dangers on both sides, or in rivers, harbours and their approaches. Coastal and channel navigation are often described by the term *pilotage*, and the boat is said to be in pilotage waters. Pilotage calls for a knowledge of charts, tide tables and other publications, and also of man-made aids to navigation such as buoys, lights, fog signals and radio aids. But first some knowledge of the earth and various units of measurement concerned with it are necessary.

Planet earth
The earth is not a perfect sphere, but can be considered such for the purposes of practical navigation. Our planet rotates from west to east and the ends of the earth's axis of spin are called the *poles*. The imaginary line midway between the poles running east-west around the earth is called the *equator*. Any straight line joining the poles is called a *meridian*, and it cuts the equator at right angles or 90 degrees (90°).

Great circle
A great circle is the largest circle that could be drawn around the earth. The equator is one example. Technically it is any circle the plane of which passes through the centre of the earth. Each meridian is half a great circle

and if one were cut right through the earth, the sphere would be divided into two equal halves. (Any other circle on the earth is called a *small circle*.) In Fig. 1 , the ribbon stretched across the globe is part of a great circle, which is the shortest distance between any two points on the earth, and in this illustration the shortest distance between New York and London. This can be important on long ocean passages, but is of only academic interest in coastal cruising.

Fig. 2 *The great circle*

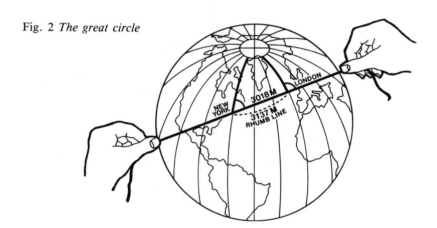

Latitude
In Fig. 3a, a line has been drawn from point A to the centre of the earth, C. The meridian through A cuts the equator at point X, and the line joining this point to the centre is also shown. The angle at the centre between these two lines is 30°, as is the angle between the lines from point B and the equator. The two places are in the Northern Hemisphere, and the latitude of both A and B is 30° north.

A line joining all the places with the same latitude is called a *parallel of latitude*, because they run east-west around the earth and are parallel to the equator and to each other. The parallels of 30° and 60° north and south of the equator are shown in the diagram. The equator makes no angle with itself, so its latitude is 0°. The angle at the centre between the equator and a line dropped from either of the poles is a right angle, so the latitudes of the poles are 90°N and 90°S respectively.

Position on the earth
In order to define the exact position of any given spot on the earth's surface it is necessary to grid the world up in some way, preferably with horizontal and vertical lines crossing at right angles. The parallels of latitude make convenient horizontal lines. The logical vertical lines to use are the meridians and these must therefore be numbered in some way.

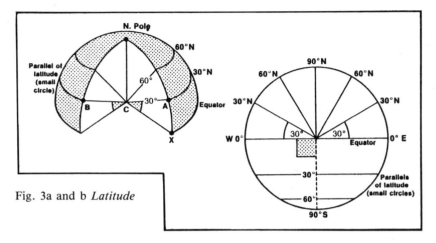

Fig. 3a and b *Latitude*

Longitude

By international agreement in 1884, the meridian through Greenwich was adopted as the zero or prime meridian. Longitude is the angular distance of a place east or west of the Greenwich meridian. Fig. 4a shows that the angle at the centre of the earth measured in the plane of the equator, between Greenwich and an arbitrary meridian to the west, is 90°. The longitude of *any* place on this meridian is therefore 90°W. East and west longitudes meet at the 180° meridian as shown in Fig. 4b.

Position by latitude and longitude

The position of any point on the earth's surface can be defined by its latitude from 0° to 90° north or south of the equator, and its longitude

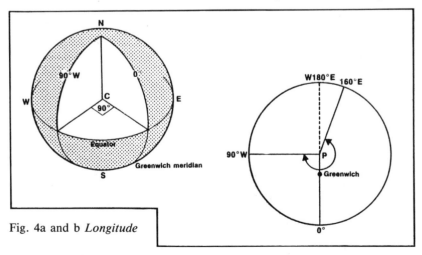

Fig. 4a and b *Longitude*

from 0° to 180° east or west of Greenwich. Both are angular measurements, and in any angular measurement there are 60 minutes of arc in a degree.

Position is given in degrees, minutes and tenths of a minute, and it is common practice to give latitude first. For example, Sydney is listed as being in latitude thirty-three degrees, fifty-two minutes south, one hundred and fifty-one degrees thirteen minutes point one east of the Greenwich meridian. This is written as 33°52′.0S, 151°13′.1E.

Latitude and longitude can be expressed in degrees, minutes and seconds of arc or angle, there being 60 seconds in a minute of arc. While this system still has certain uses, the reader may ignore it for practical pilotage purposes.

Distance and speed

Because the earth is a sphere, the distance covered on its surface when moving through one degree in any direction is the same, i.e., when moving 1/360th of a great circle. Although longitude is measured in degrees, the meridians slowly converge until they meet at a point at the pole. So the length of a degree of longitude is not constant. This is explained more fully on page 13. However, it can be seen from Fig. 3b, for example, that the distances from latitude 0° to 30° and 30° to 60° are equal in length, so the length of a degree of latitude is a constant value. To allow the navigator to convert directly from angle to distance, the nautical mile is used in navigation.

Nautical mile

A nautical or sea mile is the distance on the earth's surface represented by one minute of latitude or arc. As there are 60 minutes in a degree, so there are 60 nautical miles in one degree of latitude.

The International Nautical Mile is 1852 metres in length. Kilometres are not generally used at sea, nor was the land or statute mile often used.

The abbreviation for the sea mile is M. So, for example, twenty-eight miles is written as 28 M.

Speed at sea is measured in knots, and one knot is equal to one nautical mile per hour.

Direction

Before the navigator can take a craft from one place to another, the direction of travel between the two places must be found. On land, this sort of information is often given verbally by statements such as, 'First on the left, second on the right and you can't miss it', probably accompanied by an airy wave of the hand. However, at sea, direction must often be known more precisely. Steering a boat down the coast with plenty of landmarks in sight may be simple enough by day, but at night, in fog or thick weather there may be no reference points to be seen. In order to go in a given direction, it is necessary to refer to some datum line or fixed direction. The north-south meridian through a boat is taken as the zero or datum line and the angle in degrees measured clockwise from north is used to measure true direction.

Bearing

The direction in which a place or object lies from a vessel is called the true bearing. There are 360° in a circle, and bearings are numbered from 0° to 360°. Courses and bearings in the present-day circular notation are given in three figures, e.g., north is either zero zero zero degrees (000°) or three six zero degrees (360°). One degree to the left of north is three five nine degrees (359°). E, S, and W are zero nine zero (090°), one eight zero (180°) and two seven zero (270°) respectively.

Course and heading

The course is the direction of travel of a boat, i.e., forwards or backwards, not up and down or round and round. It is the angle measured clockwise from north between the north-south meridian through the boat and the intended direction of movement. A boat can be thrown momentarily off course by a wave, and an inexperienced helmsman may be unable to hold a steady course. Thus the boat's heading is the direction in which the bow is pointing at any given moment. The future or intended path of a vessel is called the *track*. (See also *ground track*.)

Relative bearings

Direction given with reference to the bow or fore and aft line of a boat is called a *relative bearing*. The bearings are measured clockwise from dead ahead (0° REL) through 360°, but this system is mainly used with radar and radio direction finding sets. A modification of more practical value for everyday use is called *angle on the bow*, and here the angles

Fig. 5 *Measuring true course and bearing*

Fig. 6 *Relative bearings and angle on the bow*

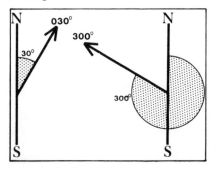

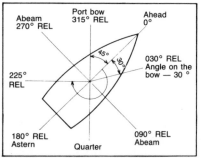

7

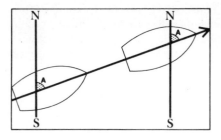

Fig. 7 *Rhumb line. Angle A is the course. This rhumb line cuts the meridians at an angle of 60°, and the boat can move along the line by steering course 060° T.*

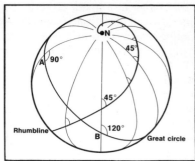

Fig. 8 *Rhumb line tracks are longer than the more direct great circle tracks.*

are measured from 0° to 180° on either side of the boat. An object might then be described as being 30° on the starboard bow (030° REL) or 10° on the port bow (350° REL). The time-tested expressions 'on the bow', 'on the beam' and 'on the quarter', without any specified number of degrees, mean respectively 45°, 90° and 135° from dead ahead. If a lookout or other person suddenly wants to call attention to an object or event sighted, these expressions or other angles on the bow are useful; for example, 'Quick, shooting star, flashing light, etc., on the port quarter'. Giving this direction as 225° REL means exactly the same thing, but try working it out in a hurry! A point to watch when using the fore and aft line as a reference is that, if the boat's heading changes, so does the relative bearing or angle on the bow of any given object.

Rhumb line
Any line that cuts all meridians at the same angle is called a *rhumb line*. This means that a boat can move along a rhumb line track by steering one constant course, assuming that there are no currents or other offsetting factors.

Equipment
The basic equipment to use for coastal navigation consists of a chart, parallel rulers, a Douglas protractor, navigational set squares or other proprietary brand instruments used for drawing courses and bearings, dividers, pencils, an eraser, a chart table, a speedometer (called a log) and a magnetic compass.

A *chart* is primarily concerned with showing the coastline and the sea. Its main purpose is to give the information necessary to get a boat safely from one place to another. Charts show prominent coastal features, navigation lights and marks, depth of water, rocks, shoals and mudflats.

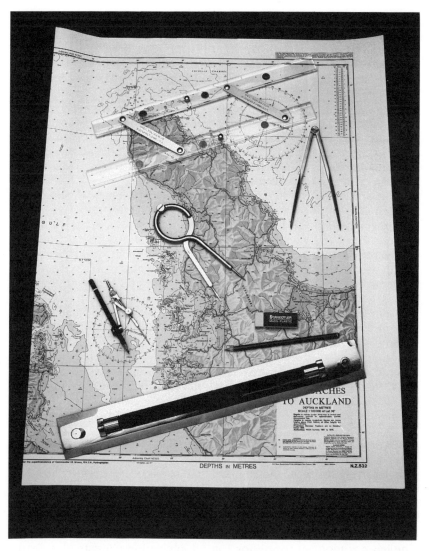

Fig. 9 *Chart and coastal navigation instruments. Top to bottom: parallel rulers, straight dividers, bow dividers, compasses, soft eraser, B or 2B pencil, roller rulers.*

A chart is different from a map because maps are primarily concerned with the land areas of the world, showing states and nations, towns and cities, mountain ranges and other features of the land.

Parallel rulers consist of two rules connected by pivotal crosspieces. They are used to draw parallel lines in draughting or chartwork. The

9

rulers can also be stepped across the face of the chart for measuring courses and bearings.

A second type of parallel rule is called a roller rule, and it has two metal wheels fitted so that it can be rolled across the surface of the chart. Either type of parallel rule is suitable. The pivotal type varies in length from roughly 30 to 50 centimetres (exactly 12, 15 and 18 inches). The long ones are good but expensive, and the shorter ones are quite suitable for the beginner. However, ensure that they have some cork discs on the underside because these give a good grip on the chart surface, which is necessary when the boat is rolling. If roller rules are chosen, ensure that they are heavier than the pivotal variety of the same length.

Dividers are used to measure distances in chart-work. Either the straight or the one-handed bow type is satisfactory, but both should be large enough to open out to at least 20 to 22 centimetres.

Pencils with B or 2B leads should be used, but no softer as they will smudge. Hard (HB) pencils can score the surface of a chart and their marks are difficult to erase.

You will need at least two good *erasers* on the chart table. One of the mysteries of the sea is the speed at which pencils and erasers disappear. Keep a few spares hidden elsewhere on the boat, such as in the bilges.

The *chart table* is probably any convenient flat surface which can be built into the hull, or perhaps the saloon table adapted for use at sea. It should be made as comfortable as possible.

The *log* in most newly-constructed boats is built into the hull, and both the boat's speed and the distance travelled register on a dial in the cockpit. How the navigator uses this information and the method of checking the log's accuracy are explained in Chapter Six.

Magnetic compasses are instruments used to indicate direction. There are two main types, a fixed and a hand bearing compass (HBC). The fixed compass is installed near the helmsman for use in steering the boat. Many brands are on sale and the navigator should be guided by a marine supplier in choosing the model best suited to his or her needs. The hand bearing compass is completely portable and is used when finding the boat's position on the coast. Both types are discussed further in Chapter Four, and the practical use of the HBC is discussed on page 82.

Books

Some of the principal Admiralty books dealing with various aspects of navigation are described here.

The Mariners' Handbook contains details of all books and publications issued by the Admiralty, including notes on charts, lights and buoyage and other information intended for the professional navigator rather than the amateur.

The *Sailing Directions* or *Admiralty Pilots* contain detailed information on ports and harbours and their approaches, local tides, currents and

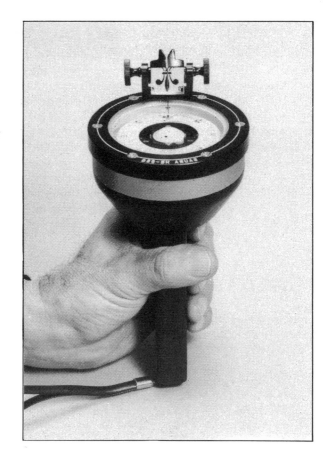

Fig. 10 *A hand
bearing compass
(HBC)*

weather. Like charts, they are kept corrected by *Notices to Mariners.*
Examples of *Admiralty Pilots* are Pacific Islands, Australia (Vols 1 to 5)
and New Zealand *Pilots*, and they are useful references for any yacht
bookshelf.

The *Admiralty List of Lights* is published in several volumes to cover
the world, and it gives details of light, light structures and fog signals.
Outside the United Kingdom, national authorities may publish similar
volumes covering their own countries, e.g., the *New Zealand Nautical
Almanac and Tide Tables.* These are essential for those who do a lot
of coastal work.

The *Admiralty Tide Tables* give tidal predictions for major and minor
ports, published in three volumes to cover the world.

The *Admiralty List of Radio Signals* is the six-volume work dealing
with all aspects of radio services available to the mariner, including coast
radio stations, radio beacons, meteorological services, radio time signals

11

and position fixing systems. However, the amateur navigator can usually find the information pertinent to his own harbour and region in locally produced publications.

The 24-hour clock

The reader will know that there are 24 hours in a day, which is divided into two 12-hour periods, each identified by using a.m. or p.m. to avoid ambiguity. However, any arithmetic using this system can be unwieldy. To illustrate this point, I would like the reader to work out what the arrival time would be for a boat that set out at 3 a.m. on a journey that would take 19 hours. The answer is 10 p.m., but how many mental steps did you have to take? Did you even have to grab a piece of paper and a pencil to do the calculation?

In navigation the day runs from midnight to midnight, i.e., from 0 to 24 hours. Time is written or expressed in four figures for hours and minutes or six figures when using hours, minutes, and seconds. For example, ten hours, fifteen minutes and six seconds would be written as 10 h 15 m 06 s. Normally a time measurement is only needed to the nearest minute, in which case this would be expressed in a less formal manner, i.e., 1015. This 24-hour clock, as it is called, is being used more and more often in places such as hospitals and in timetables, as any air traveller will know. The hours are numbered straight through, as should be clear from the following table.

1.00 a.m.	= **0100**	oh one double oh
8.30 a.m.	= **0830**	oh eight thirty
10.43 a.m.	= **1043**	ten forty-three
12.00	= **1200**	twelve hundred
1.00 p.m.	= **1300**	thirteen hundred
8.30 p.m.	= **2030**	twenty thirty
10.43 p.m.	= **2243**	twenty-two forty-three
11.59 p.m.	= **2359**	twenty-three fifty-nine

Use the suffix 'hours' if you wish, but in the context it is not necessary. After all, since when did you tell a friend that the time was 'a quarter to eleven hours'?

Now, using this notation, the earlier question can be answered by straight addition, i.e.:

Start	0300
Time taken	+ 19
Arrival time	2200

The main problem for the beginner comes when working in hours and minutes because there are 60 minutes in an hour. For example, say it is now ten o'clock. What time was it five hours thirty-seven minutes ago?

Time	10 h 00 m
	− 5 h 37 m
Time	04 h 23 m

12

The 23 minutes in the answer were found by subtracting 37 minutes from 60 minutes.

Example 1   Find the number of hours and minutes between 2.14 a.m. and 11.23 a.m.

```
  11 h 23 m
− 02 h 14 m
  09 h 09 m
```

Example 2   A boat leaves its moorings at 0837, and sails for 7 h 15 m. Find the time.

```
  0837
+ 0715
  1552
```

Example 3   Another boat departs a place at 1759, and sails for 5 h 11 m. Find the time.
Answer: 2310 (not 2270! There are only 60 minutes in an hour.)

CHARTS

The navigator needs to find the following characteristics in a chart.
   1. Countries should be easily recognisable, i.e., they should retain the same shape as they have on the globe.
   2. The parallels of latitude and meridians of longitude should be east-west and north-south lines respectively, and should cross at right angles as they do on the globe.
   3. A straight line between any two places should give the direction and distance between them. The angle at which this line cuts any meridian should give the course to steer between them, i.e., it would be a rhumb line.

Projections

The system whereby the world or areas of it are shown on a chart is called a *projection*. The problem for the chartmaker is to represent the rounded surface of the globe on the flat plane surface of a piece of paper. Regardless of the projection used, this cannot be done without some distortion or stretching.
   On the equator, a degree of latitude and a degree of longitude are the same length, i.e., 60 miles. If two ships started 60 miles apart on the equator and moved due north, they would come slowly closer together until they met at the North Pole, because here the meridians of longitude converge at a point. The distance between meridians of longitude therefore lessens, and, for example, if these two ships reached 60°N, they would be only 30 miles apart, or half the length of a degree of latitude.

The Mercator Projection

In the mid-sixteenth century, a Flemish geographer named Mercator realised that if the meridians of longitude ran vertically up and down a chart, i.e., they were parallel to each other because the length of a degree of longitude was kept constant, the length of a degree of latitude would have to be progressively increased to keep the same proportion between the two as on the globe. The effect of lengthening the latitude scale to compensate for the constant longitude scale is that the land masses are 'stretched' the closer the latitude approaches 90°. The land masses retain their shape on a Mercator projection but towards the polar regions they are larger than they are on the globe. For example, Greenland is smaller than Australia, but on a Mercator chart both countries appear to be the same size.

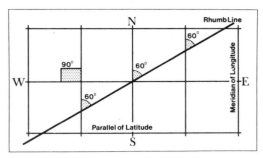

Fig. 11 *Mercator projection showing that the course to steer to go along the rhumb line is 060° T.*

The first chart to use this projection was published in 1569. Today most wall maps and coastal charts are Mercator, the main advantage as far as the navigator is concerned being that a straight line joining any two places is the rhumb line between them. The angle at which this line cuts any meridian is the course to steer to go along the line.

The gnomonic projection

Gnomonic charts (silent 'g') are used in polar regions where the Mercator latitude distortion becomes too great, and also as great circle charts. A

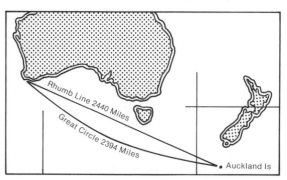

Fig. 12 *The difference between a rhumb line and a great circle on a Mercator chart*

14

straight line between any two points on the chart represents the shortest distance between the two. However, north of the equator on a Mercator Chart a great circle appears to curve to the north. The direction of curvature changes at the equator towards the south pole as shown in Fig. 12.

The chart title

Information in the chart title includes the type of projection used and the scale of the chart. More importantly, it shows whether depths and heights are given in metres or in fathoms and feet (1 fathom = 6 feet or 1.8 metres). There may be one or more 'Cautions', and as these can affect the small boat owner, they should be read carefully whenever a new chart is bought. Some harbour plans or coastal charts may be on an unfamiliar projection, but they will resemble a Mercator projection chart and can be used in all respects like one.

Scale

The natural scale of a chart is included in the title and is the ratio between the measurement on the chart and the actual distance on the surface of the earth. A large-scale chart shows a small area of the earth's surface in great detail, while a small-scale chart shows large areas such as oceans but with very much less detail. Typical natural scales in use are 1:3 500 000 for ocean charts, 1:100 000 for coastal areas and 1:18 000 for harbour plans. The largest-scale chart should always be used close to land or entering harbour because the navigator is given the maximum information about lighthouses, buoys and beacons, depths of water and navigational hazards such as rocks, reefs and shoals.

Chart symbols

The space available on charts is limited, so a great deal of information is given in abbreviations or as symbols. These are standardised all over the world because of the work of the International Hydrographic Organisation (IHO), so, no matter in what country the chart has been produced, any seafarer can understand and use it. In New Zealand the information is contained in booklet NZ 201 (INT 1), and in Australia the Admiralty booklet 5011 (INT 1) is used.

Many abbreviations are self-evident, as shown by those giving information on the nature of the seabed, i.e.: S   sand; M   mud; Sh   shells; St   stones; Sn   shingle; R   rock.

Additional information is given by combining adjectives with the above, e.g.: c   coarse; so   soft; f   fine; gy   grey; sm   small; bl   black.

So fine sand would be 'fS' and small shells would be 'sm Sh'. My favourite is 'bl Gl Oz', i.e., black globigerina ooze. No, I don't know what it means either, but I like it.

Heights are given to the nearest whole metre, but depths of less than

1	*h*	Hour	†9	*fm*	Fathom(s)
2	*min*	Minute (of time)	11	M	Sea Mile(s)
3	*sec,s*	Second (of time)	12	*kn*	Knot(s)
4	*m*	Metre(s)	12a	*t*	Ton
4a	*dm*	Decimetre(s)	13	Lat	Latitude
4b	*cm*	Centimetre(s)	14	Long	Longitude
4c	*mm*	Millimetre(s)	19	Ht	Height
5	*km*	Kilometre(s)	20	°	Degree
†6	*in.*	Inch(s)	21	'	Minute (of arc)
7	*ft*	Foot; feet	22	"	Second (of arc)
†8	*yd*	Yard(s)	23	No	Number

Fig. 13 (left) *Chart symbols: Units*

Fig. 14 (below left) *Chart symbols: Landmarks*

Fig. 15 (below) *Local facilities*

1	⚓Building ⊙Hotel	Examples of landmarks
2	⚓ BUILDING ⊙ HOTEL WATER TOWER	Examples of conspicuous landmarks
3.1	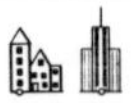	Pictorial symbols (in true position)
3.2	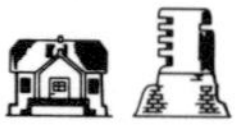	Sketches, Views (out of position)
4	(30)	Height of top of a structure above plane of reference for heights
5	(30)	Height of structure above ground level

KEY TO SPECIAL SYMBOLS OF INTEREST TO SMALL CRAFT	
	Slipway for small craft
	Yacht berth
	Visitors' mooring
	Visitors' berth
	Water tap
	Fuel
	Public Landing
P	Public Car Park
	Parking for boats/trailers
WC	Toilets
	Public Telephone
	Yacht or Sailing Club

31 metres are shown in metres and decimetres, e.g., 16_7 is 16.7 metres. Other useful abbreviations are given in Chapter Three.

The chartmakers are responding to the needs of the boating public by including such information as the table of special symbols of interest to small craft, shown in Fig. 15, on many harbour charts and plans.

Plotting latitude and longitude

If the latitude and longitude of a point are known, the position can be plotted on a chart by one of two methods.

1. Place one edge of a parallel ruler along one of the parallels of latitude printed on the chart and move the ruler until one edge passes through the latitude of the place, as shown by the latitude scale on the side of the chart. Pencil in the latitude line. Now line up the ruler with a meridian of longitude and move the ruler across the chart until one edge is through the correct longitude. Pencil in the point at which this

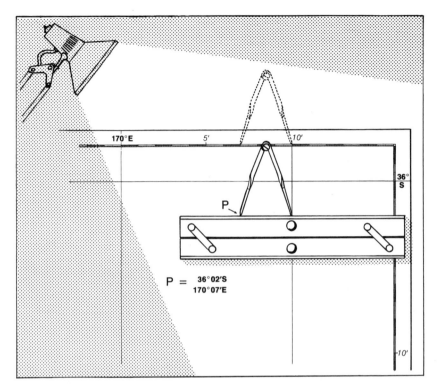

Fig. 16 *Plotting a point by latitude and longitude*

edge crosses the latitude line; this is the required position.

2. Line the ruler up on the correct latitude, as explained above. With the dividers, measure the distance at the top or bottom of the chart from the nearest meridian to the required longitude. Lay this off along the latitude line, as shown in Fig. 16.

The edge of the ruler facing the main source of light should be used, as the other edge will cast a shadow. This is important at night on a dimly lit chart table, when trying to use the shadow-casting edge may result in the latitude scale being read incorrectly. Anyway, why make life difficult?

Measuring distance on a chart

Remember that one minute of latitude is equal to one nautical mile. Distance on a chart is measured by opening a pair of dividers until the points are on the two places in question, and moving the dividers to the nearest side of the chart to find the distance on the *latitude scale*. The latitude scale is printed up and down each side of a chart, as shown in

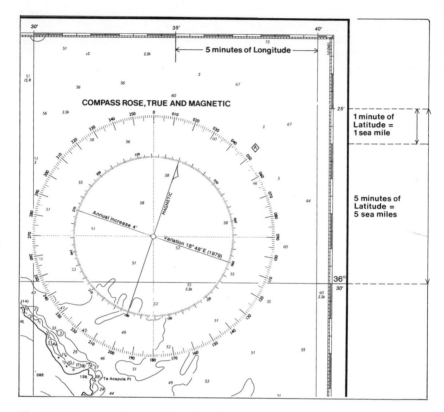

Fig. 17 *Distance scale on a Mercator chart*

Fig. 17. If the dividers cover, say, 6 minutes of latitude, the distance being measured is 6 nautical miles. On most charts, and in Fig. 17, each mile is subdivided into tenths, so it is usual to measure and express distances in miles and decimals of a mile, e.g., 6.3 M is six point three miles. Older charts sometimes had a second distance scale given in thousands of yards. Metric charts may give an equivalent scale in thousands of metres for the sake of convenience, but this is not to be confused with measuring distance in kilometres.

If a long distance is being measured, the dividers should be set at a convenient distance apart (say 5 or 10 miles) and stepped off along the line joining the two points. I said earlier that on a Mercator chart of the world, Greenland and Australia appeared to be the same size. If they are measured very carefully, using the latitude scale horizontally opposite each country, you will find that Greenland is the smaller of the two.

One last point: the longitude scale that runs across the top and bottom of a chart must *never* be used to measure distance.

The compass rose

Fig. 17 shows a compass rose, used for measuring courses or bearings. The outer circle of figures indicates true directions, measured from 0° to 360° clockwise from north. Several roses are usually overprinted at convenient places on the chart.

Most true compass roses have a smaller inner circle called the *magnetic ring*, used for measuring magnetic direction. Their use is fully explained in Chapter Four.

Measuring courses

One edge of the parallel rulers should be aligned so that it joins the boat's starting point and the destination. Then step the rulers over to the nearest rose so that either outer edge goes through the centre spot on the rose (Fig. 18). The reading on the outside circle where the same edge of the ruler cuts it is the true course between the two points.

The procedure is reversed when laying off a course from a given starting point. Line one edge of the rulers from the centre point of the rose so that it cuts the outer ring at the desired course or bearing. Move either of the outer edges to the start point on the chart, and draw in

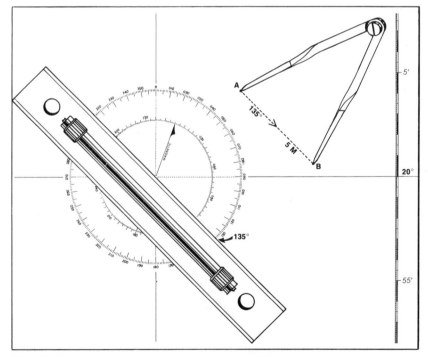

Fig. 18 *Course and distance from A to B is 135°T, 5 miles*

19

the course/bearing line. I know, I know — the stupid rulers start to walk right off the chart, miles from where you want them. If this happens, swing one ruler right around on the pivots, holding the other rule firm, and start again from there.

You will soon get the hang of it, and with a bit of practice they can be walked from one corner of a chart to any other corner.

Combination plotting instruments

Attempts have been made to combine the functions of parallel rulers, compass rose and dividers in the one instrument. Most of these have been derived from air navigation plotters designed during World War II for use by fighter pilots in cramped cockpits, so are particularly useful in small craft. Fig. 19 shows one example, which is suitable for general chartwork, and for changing true to magnetic directions to find compass courses to steer.

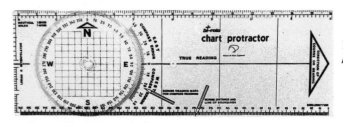

Fig. 19 *Chart protractor*

Chart corrections

The moment a new chart comes off the printing press, it starts going out of date. New lights may be built or colours and characteristics changed, buoys may break away from their moorings in storms and new hazards to navigation are discovered. Thus a chart either lacks certain information, or some of the information on the chart is outdated if it is not corrected.

Changes are issued weekly by naval authorities in each country in booklet form and these are called *Notices to Mariners* (Fig. 20). Major chart agents are usually required by contract to keep their stocks of new charts corrected and up to date with the latest *Notices*, although in Australia a new chart will be accompanied by a correction slip listing all the *Notices* outstanding. The navigator must then insert these corrections on the chart. Small chart stockists such as the local marine hardware store may not be required to do this, and the reader should be aware that any charts bought from such sources may not have been corrected for weeks or even months.

Permanent corrections such as new lights established or buoys moved should be entered on the chart in violet ink and the year and number of the correction noted on the bottom left opposite the heading 'Small

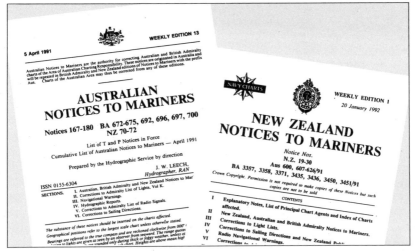

Fig. 20 *Notices to Mariners*

Corrections' (Fig. 21). When changes are only temporary, for example, if a buoy has been taken ashore for painting, the notices have a 'T' after the number. Temporary changes are put on the chart in pencil so that they can be erased when the change is remedied.

Chart agents do not have to enter 'T' notices on their charts. However, each weekly edition contains a list of all temporary notices still in force, with a précis of each one. By checking this list, the navigator can see if any are in force for the particular area.

Preliminary notices give advance information on coming changes; for example, a new lighthouse may take a year or more to build. A preliminary *Notice* will be published, telling the mariner that it is under construction. When it is completed, a permanent *Notice* will be issued and then the light is inked on the chart.

Well, that's the theory. I know that not all small boat owners, for whatever good reasons, manage to keep their charts corrected and up to date. Nevertheless, all yachtsmen, wherever they may be, should skim through the temporary *Notices* every two or three weeks. Most yacht and power boat clubs make them readily available to members. As to the inked corrections, if readers are unable to keep up with these, they should at least buy a new chart of their local area at the start of each season.

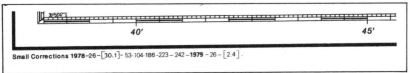

Fig. 21 *Corrections are listed on the bottom corner of a chart*

Chapter Two
Tides

The periodic rises and falls in the level of the sea in a harbour or around a coastline are called *tides*. The sea level rises until it reaches a maximum height, called high water (HW) or high tide, then falls to a minimum level called low water (LW) or low tide, so a tide is the up and down or vertical movement of water. The horizontal movement of water that results from these changes in sea levels is called *tidal stream* or *tidal flow*. The movement of water usually associated with the incoming tide leading to high water is called the *flood stream* and the movement of water associated with the outgoing tide leading to low water is called the *ebb stream*. The period of time at high or low water during which there is no discernible change in the vertical level of the water is called the *stand* of the tide. During the period between alternate ebb and flood streams when there is no horizontal flow, it is said to be *slack* water. The range of the tide is the vertical distance the sea level rises between LW and the succeeding HW, or falls between HW and the next LW.

Causes

In understanding the general causes of tides, it is useful to refresh one's memory on the nature of a wave. Although the waves in a body of water such as a lake or the sea may travel with considerable speed, the water itself simply rises and falls. When the wave reaches shallow water, the lower part is slowed, the front of the wave steepens and the faster-moving top curls over, finally breaks and flows in over the beach. This may give the erroneous impression that the water of the wave actually moves along

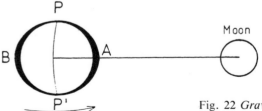

Fig. 22 *Gravitational pull of the moon*

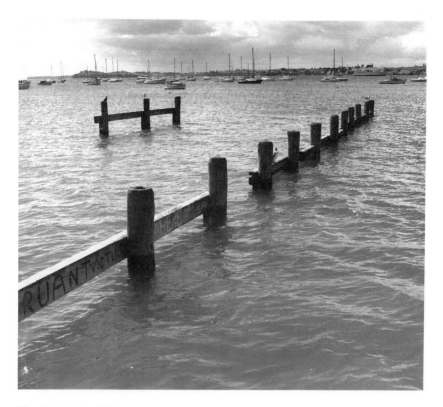

Fig. 23 *Spring high water*

with the wave. The other optical illusion is that when the tide comes in and goes out, the water appears to move backwards and forwards across the sand in a horizontal direction. It does, but only because the level of water in the bay is rising or falling.

Full tidal theory is quite complex and a thorough understanding is not needed by the average yachtsman. For our purposes, tides are caused by the gravitational forces of the moon and the sun. Although the sun is the larger of the two, the moon is much closer to the earth and has the greater effect.

In Fig. 22, it is assumed that the globe is entirely covered by water. The moon is directly overhead and therefore closest to point A on the earth.

The gravitational pull of the moon is strongest at this point and is acting on both earth and water, but only the water is free to move. A build-up of water is formed, giving high water at A. Point B, which is diametrically opposite A, is the most distant point on the earth from the moon. Here

23

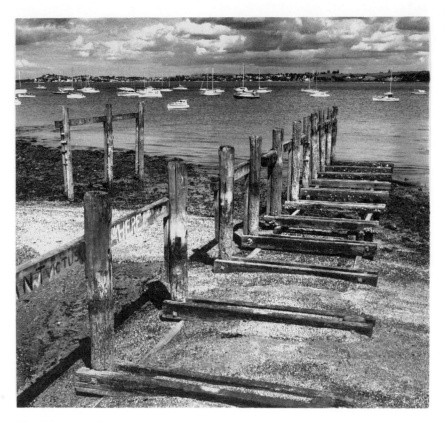

Fig. 24 *Spring low water*

a second build-up or high water is formed; clearly this cannot be due to the moon's gravity, since the pull is in the wrong direction. In effect, being farthest from the moon, this high water is due to a comparative lack of the moon's gravitational pull at B. There will be low water at the meridians of longitude P and P¹ which are halfway between A and B.

As the earth rotates on its axis, the two high waters or tide waves move across the earth's surface. When the earth has rotated so that A has arrived at B and B at A, each will have a second high water. The earth spins once around its axis every 24 hours, so there are usually two high waters and two low waters at a place each day. In the open seas the general rise in level as this wave, caused by the tide-producing force of the moon, passes, is spread over such a large area that it is unnoticed by any vessel.

The sun has only 43% of the effect of the moon but its attractive force causes another set of high waters beneath it. Look at Fig. 25, which shows the situation at new moon. The tide-producing forces of the sun and moon are reinforcing each other. Approximately fifteen days later at full moon, when the earth is between the sun and the moon, the two again act along the same line. On both these occasions, i.e., about twice a month, spring tides occur and they give the highest high waters and the lowest low waters. Due to the effects of friction and inertia, spring tides occur one or two days after full or new moon.

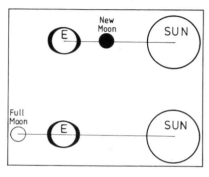

Fig. 25 *New moon*

Fig. 26 *Tide-raising force of the moon in its first or last quarter*

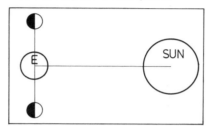

When the moon is in its first or last quarter, its tide-raising force is exerted at right angles to that of the sun, as shown in Fig. 26. The resultant tides, called neap tides, are the smallest of the month. The high waters do not rise to the same level as those at springs; on the other hand, the low waters do not fall as far. As tidal streams are generally directly related to the rise and fall of the tides, they will be strongest at springs and weakest at neaps.

This explanation of tides' general causes assumes that the earth is completely covered with water and that the tide waves caused by the moon and the sun are free to circle the globe. Even though the continents and land masses get in the way, any large body of water will respond to the tide-producing forces of the moon and sun. The Atlantic, Pacific and Indian Oceans can be regarded as separate masses of water and large tides are generated in each. In contrast, the tides in the land-locked Mediterranean Sea are quite small. On approaching land, the tide wave may be forced to divert by the underwater topography or the land mass itself. For example, in the United Kingdom, the wave divides at Lands End and part travels up the English Channel, arriving at Dover about seven hours later. The remainder moves up the Irish coast and finally into the North Sea.

Local tides

As most places have two high waters and two low waters every 24 hours, the interval between one LW and the next HW or the HW and succeeding LW is approximately six hours. This interval is called the *duration* of the tide. However, the characteristics of the tides can vary quite widely from port to port and from region to region. For example, some parts of the Pacific Ocean have only one high water and one low water a day. Southampton in the United Kingdom differs from other south coast ports in having double tides, i.e. four high and four low waters each day. Many harbours have a tidal range of two or three metres but due to local sea bed and coastal features, some may have tides with ranges from nine to twelve metres. Darwin, St Helier in France and the port of Bristol are examples of these.

Tidal streams

Although tidal streams are caused by the tides, the navigator should not assume that slack water at a port occurs at the time of high or low water. In many places, the periods of flood and ebb stream do coincide with those of the rising and falling tide, and slack water in the harbour occurs during the stands of the tides. But, for example, around the coasts of New Zealand and offshore in the English Channel, the change in direction of a tidal stream seldom coincides with the time of high or low water by the shore.

To understand how streams are influenced by local conditions, let us compare two tidal basins. The first has access to the sea by a wide opening, the second has a narrow and constricted entrance. In the first case, the tide wave on approaching the coast has direct access to the basin. The process of filling or emptying it keeps pace with the change in sea level and it is almost completed at the time of slack water outside. The speed of the tidal stream through the opening will be greatest when the height of the tide inside is changing most rapidly, i.e., about halfway between HW and LW.

In the second case, the narrow entrance does not allow the basin to fill or empty very quickly, so on a flood tide the level of water outside the basin is higher than the level inside. Even when the tide has turned on the coast, the level inside is lower than that outside, and water keeps flowing in. The speed of the tidal stream through the entrance will be greatest when there is the maximum difference between the two water levels, i.e., at the times of HW and LW on the coast. The tidal stream into the basin will not reverse direction until the water levels inside and outside are the same. In some places this common level is not reached until mid-tide, and at these places the tidal stream will flood until three hours after high water and ebb until three hours after low water. In practice this situation is found in narrow bays and long channels. The first case explained above occurs on open coasts and in wide-mouthed bays and bights.

Although tidal streams are a direct effect of tides, they may not act in unison. In these cases it is better to drop the terms 'ebb' and 'flood' and to talk about the general direction of a particular tidal stream, i.e., a north-going stream or an east-going stream, and so on. Winds are named according to the direction whence they come. A northerly wind blows from the north. The direction of a tidal stream is that in which it moves; its course, if you like. Its speed is given in knots.

TIDE TABLES

The times of high and low water and heights of the tide can be found from one of the sets of tide tables available at any ships' chandler and often from the daily newspaper. Tables produced by local harbour authorities contain detailed information on a particular port and nearby coastal areas. National marine authorities publish tables each year with predictions for all their large and small ports. The *Admiralty Tide Tables*, published annually in three volumes, give world-wide coverage.

General layout

The general layout of the *Australian National Tide Tables* and *New Zealand Tide Tables* is exactly the same. Part 1 consists of daily predictions for major ports (called *standard ports*) given in the following form:

0241	1.2
0850	3.4
1502	1.4
2120	3.2

The first column gives the times of the tides on a given day and the second column gives the heights in metres above chart datum. So in this example the predicted times and heights of HW are 0850, 3.4 m and 2120, 3.2 m. Those of LW are 0241, 1.2 m and 1502, 1.4 m. The official standard time at the port is used in these predictions and is given in the heading of the table. This should be checked, because an hour may have to be added if summer time is being kept.

The actual depth of water at high or low tide can be found by adding the predicted height to any sounding (depth) given on the chart, e.g.:

Chart depth	10.2 m
Height of HW	+ 3.4 m
Depth of water at 0850	13.6 m

The range of the tide is the total rise or fall in water level between one high water and the preceding or next low water. The duration is the time elapsing between high water and low water or vice versa, e.g.:

Predicted time of HW	0850
Predicted time of LW	0241
Duration of the tide	0609

Height of HW	3.4
Height of LW	1.2
Range	2.2

Secondary ports
Tidal information is listed for some 300 ports or places in Australia and over 600 in the United Kingdom. Any set of tables listing all these with full tidal details would be both bulky and expensive. The majority are given in Part II of the *Tables* and although this section is entitled 'Secondary Ports', many are important and busy harbours. The predictions for each place are given as time and height differences to be applied to the times and heights of high water and low water at a specified standard port on the same day. This is not too difficult, but there are some pitfalls. An explanation of finding the times and heights of tide at New Zealand secondary ports is given in Appendix Two.

Accuracy of the tables
The information given for standard ports is based on many years' observation of the actual tides and is reliable under average meteorological conditions. The predictions for some of the more remote secondary ports are based on more limited data and should be treated with some reserve.

Differences between the predicted and actual tides can be caused by barometric pressure and wind. A persistently low barometric pressure will mean a rise in sea level and a high pressure will tend to depress it. A change of 34 millibars can mean a height difference of about 0.3 m. A strong wind will tend to raise the sea level in the direction in which it is blowing. A constant onshore wind tends to pile up water so that both the high and low waters are higher than predicted; an offshore wind may mean that the tides are lower than predicted. A strong wind may also cause differences between the predicted and actual times of high and low water.

The readers may be thinking that this is all fine, but how are they supposed to work out the differences between actual and predicted tides? By and large, this is impossible. The moral here is that the yachtsman should *never* navigate his or her boat in just enough water to clear the keel. Always allow a margin for error of about a metre in depth. In rough weather the troughs of the big waves are below normal sea level and this margin should be doubled.

The Rule of Twelfths
The approximate height of tide at times other than high water or low water can be found by using the Rule of Twelfths. The tide does not rise and fall at a uniform rate; the maximum change in height usually occurs at mid-tide. There is relatively little change in the hour on either

side of high and low water. Thus the Rule states that the rise or fall is 1/12 of the range in the first and sixth hours, 2/12 in the second and fifth and 3/12 in the third and fourth hours.

For example, let us assume that LW is at 1000, 1.0 m and HW 1600, 3.4 m.

HW	1600		3.4
LW	1000		1.0
Duration	0600	Range	2.4

One-twelfth of 2.4 is 0.2, so the hourly change in height is equal to:

Time	Hourly change	Total change	Height of tide
1000 LW			1.0
1100 1/12	0.2	0.2	1.2
1200 2/12	0.4	0.6	1.6
1300 3/12	0.6	1.2	2.2
1400 3/12	0.6	1.8	2.8
1500 2/12	0.4	2.2	3.2
1600 1/12	0.2	2.4	3.4 HW

The Rule works on the assumption that the duration of the tide is exactly 6 hours. In the example above, the range is a convenient 2.4 m, which makes the division into twelfths easy. In practice, the duration will vary between about five and seven hours and the range will not be exactly divisible by twelve. Nevertheless, by working to the nearest 0.1 m, the result obtained should be accurate enough for the yachtsman's purposes. If the duration is outside the limits given above, the rule will be inaccurate.

Chart datum

Due to the tides, the level of the sea and therefore the depth of water is constantly changing. As only one depth (sounding) can be printed on a chart for each place, there must be a margin for safety by ensuring that the depth shown is a minimum. A boat owner who anchored in a bay in a charted depth of 2 metres only to go aground because the depth was 1 metre on his arrival could be justifiably annoyed.

Soundings are given below a low water level called *chart datum*. On the older fathom charts, this was usually the level of mean low water springs (MLWS). Occasionally the tide fell a little lower, which meant that the depth of water was slightly less than that shown on the chart. To overcome this problem, the new metric charts use a theoretical level called lowest astronomical tide (LAT). This is the lowest tidal level that can be predicted under average meteorological conditions and with any combination of sun, moon and earth. *Thus chart datum is defined as being a level below which the tide will seldom fall.* The height of the

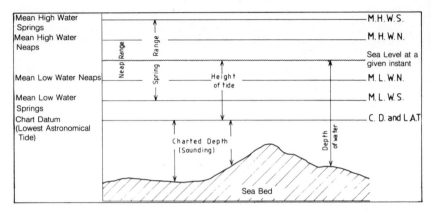

Fig 27. *Tidal levels*

tide at any moment is the height of the sea surface above chart datum. The depth of water at any moment can be found by adding the height of tide to the sounding given on the chart.

Tidal stream information

Tidal stream arrows may be shown at various points on coastal charts. These indicate the general direction of the flood and ebb streams with the average rate in knots. The difference between them — and a good memory aid — is that the *flood* stream arrow has the *feathers*.

More accurate information is given at points that show tidal diamonds. Each is identified by a letter and tidal flow data for all the diamonds are given in one table. The direction and rate in knots at springs and neaps are shown for 6 hours on either side of HW at a nearby standard port.

Fig. 29 shows a diamond marked B and information referring to HW at Auckland. The latitudes and longitudes of the four diamonds in the table are shown. Six hours before HW the direction at B is 225°T. The spring rate is 0′.3 and the neap 0′.2.

For example, this is how to find the tidal stream at B at 1230 on a day when the HW spring tide at Auckland is at 1030. First find the interval:

Time of HW Auckland	1030
Required time	1230
Interval	0200 after HW

From Fig. 29: Direction 020°; Rate 1′.0.

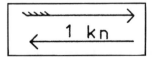

Fig. 28 *Tidal stream arrows*

30

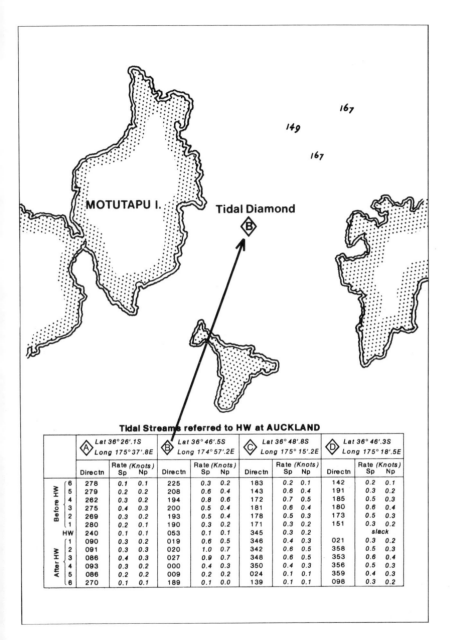

MOTUTAPU I.

Tidal Diamond

167
149
167

Tidal Streams referred to HW at AUCKLAND

		(A) Lat 36°26'.1S Long 175°37'.8E	Rate (Knots) Sp	Np	(B) Lat 36°46'.5S Long 174°57'.2E	Rate (Knots) Sp	Np	(C) Lat 36°48'.8S Long 175°15'.2E	Rate (Knots) Sp	Np	(D) Lat 36°46'.3S Long 175°18'.5E	Rate (Knots) Sp	Np
		Directn	Sp	Np	Directn	Sp	Np	Directn	Sp	Np	Directn	Sp	Np
Before HW	6	278	0.1	0.1	225	0.3	0.2	183	0.2	0.1	142	0.2	0.1
	5	279	0.2	0.2	208	0.6	0.4	143	0.6	0.4	191	0.3	0.2
	4	262	0.3	0.2	194	0.8	0.6	172	0.7	0.5	185	0.5	0.3
	3	275	0.4	0.3	200	0.5	0.4	181	0.6	0.4	180	0.6	0.4
	2	269	0.3	0.2	193	0.5	0.4	178	0.5	0.3	173	0.5	0.3
	1	280	0.2	0.1	190	0.3	0.2	171	0.3	0.2	151	0.3	0.2
HW		240	0.1	0.1	053	0.1	0.1	345	0.3	0.2	slack		
After HW	1	090	0.3	0.2	019	0.6	0.5	346	0.4	0.3	021	0.3	0.2
	2	091	0.3	0.3	020	1.0	0.7	342	0.6	0.5	358	0.5	0.3
	3	086	0.4	0.3	027	0.9	0.7	348	0.6	0.5	353	0.6	0.4
	4	093	0.3	0.2	000	0.4	0.3	350	0.4	0.3	356	0.5	0.3
	5	086	0.2	0.2	009	0.2	0.2	024	0.1	0.1	359	0.4	0.3
	6	270	0.1	0.1	189	0.1	0.0	139	0.1	0.1	098	0.3	0.2

Fig. 29 *Tidal stream information*

Chapter Three
Aids to Coastal Navigation

LIGHTS AND LIGHTHOUSES

Lights are essential aids to navigation at night. The most powerful act as homing beacons for vessels making a landfall at the end of an ocean passage.

Lighthouses are most often the well-known tall white buildings placed on headlands near the entrance to large harbours or on offshore islands. They also serve as useful navigation marks by day. Lighthouses close to one another on the same stretch of coastline may be different shapes and painted with stripes or squares for ease of identification. They will usually show a white light that is visible at twenty to thirty miles, but to avoid confusion each will have different characteristics which are described below.

Closer to harbour, lights are less powerful. They may be placed on top of any structure, ranging from a small iron framework to a lighthouse and will be visible at about ten miles. Some lights are white but others may be red or green. This use of colours helps ensure that no one light will be mistaken for any other.

Lighted buoys and beacons are placed in harbours and harbour entrances to mark the safe channels and to show hidden dangers. Because of the large number of such marks, some lights may be orange, yellow, or violet. Some colours may be used for specific purposes; for example, red lights mark the port hand side of a channel. This use of colours is explained further in the section on buoys and beacons (page 37).

Light characteristics

The lights used as aids to navigation are regulated so that they either shine continuously or operate in some form of regular cycle.

The mode of operation of any light is called its *characteristic*. The three basic characteristics are given below, together with the abbreviation for each.

F	Fixed	A continuous steady light
Fl	Flashing	A light that shows a single flash at regular intervals. The length of each flash is shorter than the length of darkness that follows.
Oc	Occulting	An occultation is a period of darkness. Hence this term describes a light that is cut off or eclipsed at regular intervals. The duration of light is longer than that of the darkness that follows.

As a guide, a flashing light will shine for one second and switch off for two to three seconds in each cycle, i.e., it flashes approximately 15 to 20 times a minute. This rate is varied to give three more distinctive characteristics.

Q	Quick Flashing	A light that flashes 50 to 60 times per minute
VQ	Very Quick Flashing	A light that flashes 100 or 120 times each minute
L Fl	Long Flashing	A light that shows a long flash of not less than 2 seconds' duration

Other characteristics are formed by combining a number of flashes or occultations (eclipses) into groups. The number in each group is given in brackets after the abbreviation, e.g.:

Fl (3)	Group Flashing, three	A light showing at regular intervals a group of three flashes followed by a longer period of darkness
Oc (2)	Group Occulting, two	A steady light with a group of two sudden eclipses at regular intervals
VQ (3)	Group Very Quick Flashing, three	A light showing at regular intervals a group of three very quick flashes followed by a longer period of darkness

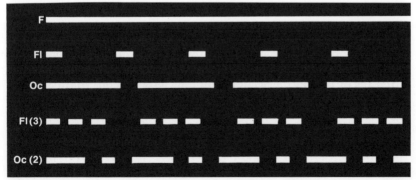

Fig. 30 *Light characteristics*

An isophase light is one in which the durations of light and darkness are equal. For example, the abbreviation 'Iso 6 sec' means that three seconds of light are followed by a three-second eclipse. The notation 'Mo' stands for Morse code. 'Mo(A)' on a chart means that the light shows a continual series of a short flash followed by a long one, as in the Morse letter A. An alternating light shows changes of colour on the same bearing. Thus 'Al WG' is a fixed light showing first a white and then a green light, and so on.

There are other possible combinations of the various characteristics discussed above, but the abbreviations are usually self-evident. The yachtsman should find that the majority of lights will fall into the categories given in the text.

Colour

The following abbreviations are used when describing the colours of lights: red (R), green (G), Orange (Y), yellow (Y), blue (Bu), and violet (Vi). If no colour abbreviation is given on the chart, the light is assumed to be white. However, if there is a combination of colours as in an alternating light, and one of them is white, W is used. The following list should make this clear.

F	A fixed white light
FG	A fixed green light
Q	A quick flashing white light
QR	A quick flashing red light
FL(2)	A white light, group flashing two
Fl(3)Y	A yellow light, group flashing three
OcR	An occulting red light
2 FR (vert)	Two fixed red lights placed vertically one above the other
Al WRG	A steady light changing colour in the sequence white, red, green

Period

The length of time between the first flash or eclipse in one cycle of a light to the beginning of the next cycle is called the *period* of the light. The notation 'Fl 15 sec' describes a white light that flashes once every 15 seconds.

'Fl(3)R 10 sec' indicates a red light that shows groups of three flashes followed by a longer period of darkness, each cycle taking 10 seconds. In line with the policy of shortening light descriptions on charts, the chartmakers have agreed that the abbreviation for seconds on new editions will be 's'. The two light descriptions I have just given will therefore become Fl 15 s and Fl(3)R 10 s. A close scrutiny of any chart will show that chartmakers put full stops in abbreviations when they feel like it and leave them out when they don't.

The navigator now has all the information needed for the positive identification of any light — its colour, characteristics and period. The last named is as important as the other features and once a light has been tentatively identified by characteristics and colour, the period should be timed. Naturally using a watch for the purpose is best, but with a little practice, periods of up to thirty seconds can be timed quite accurately by counting aloud 'one potato, two potato . . .' and so on.

Positive recognition is essential because there is a tendency for the navigator to assume that the light that comes over the horizon *must* be the one he or she is looking for. Especially in rough weather, the relief of sighting something, anything, can make the navigator's mind play tricks by convincing them that what the light is doing is what they think it should be doing. The colour, characteristics, and period should be ascertained first, and then the chart should be checked to ensure that the navigator is seeing the right light. If not, find out what light is there. The result may be horrifying.

Arcs of visibility

Coastal lights are screened so that they shine to seaward and not over the land behind. These *arcs of visibility* are often shown on charts, as in Fig. 31, but they are not intended to indicate the distance at which the light can be seen. The arc can be described by giving the limits as bearings from seaward, i.e., as seen from a boat that is under way. Thus a boat out to the east of a light has to look in a westerly direction to see it. This is also shown in the diagram; the light is visible from a bearing of 270°T through north to 045°T.

Fig. 31 *Arc of visibility*

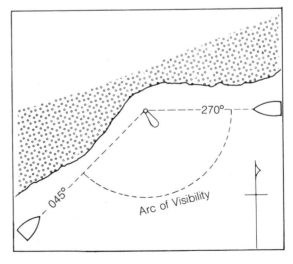

Height

The height of a light is measured above the level of mean high water springs and is included in the description on the chart. The notation 'Fl 15 s 32 m' shows that the light is 32 metres above MHWS. On older charts the heights are given in feet. In general, the higher a light the further it can be seen and this information is used in finding position, as explained in Chapter 6.

Visibility range

The distance at which a light can be seen is called its range and is given in the description on the chart. Thus 'Fl 10 s 82 m 22 M' means that the range of this light is 22 miles when seen from a height of eye of 4.5 metres above sea level in good visibility (see page 90). On modern charts where heights and depths are in metres, the visibility is given as a *nominal range*. This is the distance from which the light will be seen when the visibility is 10 miles and is independent of height of eye. For practical purposes the reader can take it that in clear weather and whatever the type of chart used, the lights will be in sight at the stated range.

The more powerful lights work on the principle of the light being concentrated into a strong beam by means of a series of lenses. The beam is rotated mechanically and is seen by a vessel offshore as a brilliant flash as the beam sweeps past. The speed of rotation is adjusted to give the light the required period. In very clear conditions the beam can be seen sweeping across the horizon when the light itself is still below it. This *loom*, as it is called, is visible at a greater distance than the charted range. The beam may also be reflected from a layer of light cloud and sighted before either the loom or the light. Because of this effect I once saw a 36-mile light at over 70 miles, but this was unusual. Despite what I have just said, if the navigator needs to use a 20-mile light as a navigation mark on the way past, he would be wise to steer a course that takes the boat no more than 16 or 17 miles off.

Some lighthouses and light beacons are fitted with fog signals that operate automatically when visibility is reduced. There are several types of fog signal, and an abbreviation for the instrument fitted in a particular light structure is given at the end of the description of the light, e.g., Fl 10 s 45 m 15 M Horn. An explanation of the various types of fog signals and the abbreviations for each are given in Chapter 10.

Sector lights

Some lights are screened to show different colours over different arcs but they usually retain the same characteristic when seen from any direction. In general a red light shows over any sector containing hidden dangers such as a rock or reef, while a white light indicates safe water or a channel. Occasionally three colours may be used and the chart must be inspected to find out why there are a number of sectors, each with its own colour. The sectors are dotted in on the chart as shown in Fig. 32. If any light is blocked from view to a vessel approaching from a given direction, that sector will be shown with the word 'obscured'. The range of the coloured light will usually be less than that of the white one, and this is indicated in the abbreviated description. For example, Fl WR 8 s 2 m 7/4 M indicates that in the white sector the light is visible for 7 miles and in the red 4 miles.

The division between arcs is indistinct in some older lights. The one constant colour as seen from a vesssel shows that it is in a given sector, but a change from one colour to another does not mean that the vessel is precisely on the dividing line between the two sectors as printed on the chart. However, new lights may be fitted with modern optical systems that give accurate sector boundaries. The navigator can experience an abrupt colour change with a lateral movement of 1.5 metres at just under three miles from the light, i.e., by merely crossing from one side of the boat to the other. These high-intensity beam or 'directional' lights are being used to mark narrow channels, especially in bar harbours, where the light is just swivelled to show safe water as the bar shifts.

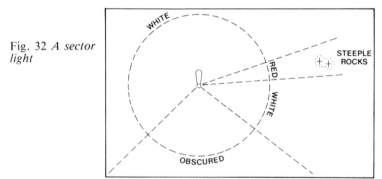

Fig. 32 *A sector light*

BUOYAGE SYSTEMS

Buoys and beacons

Buoys are floating marks anchored to the sea bed and beacons are fixed wood or metal marks built onshore, on rocks or in shallow water. They show the respective sides of deep water channels, a hidden danger or the limits of underwater hazards such as shoals, and may indicate that certain areas are used for special purposes. The five basic shapes — conical or cone, can-shaped, spherical, pillar, and spar — are shown in Fig. 33. By day the shape and colour of a buoy indicates its purpose. At night the colour and characteristic of any light that may be fitted to the buoy do the same thing. Topmarks are shapes fitted to the tops of buoys or beacons that give further information about channels or dangers. Topmarks can be a cone, a can, a cross, or a sphere.

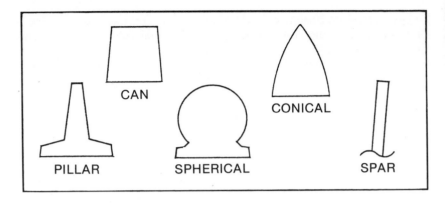

Fig. 33 *The five basic buoy shapes in the lateral system*

Prior to 1980 there was no single international system of buoyage. Coastal sailors grew accustomed to their own national systems but problems arose if they sailed into foreign waters and came across equally foreign buoyage. Most Commonwealth countries used what was called the lateral system whereas many European nations used the cardinal system.

If a deep water channel is marked with buoys on both sides it is reasonably obvious that a vessel should pass between the two lines of buoys. Inspection of the chart will also show the reason for the buoys' presence. However a problem arises if an unexpected and uncharted buoy suddenly appears ahead of a boat. The navigator must know on which side to pass the buoy to stay in deep water. If the safe thing to do is to leave the buoy on the starboard side of the boat when going in one direction then it must be on the port side when going in the opposite direction.

The principle of the lateral system is that the shape and colour of a buoy show on which side of the boat it should be kept when going into harbour. It works well in this situation, but the buoys can be ambiguous and dangerous if trying to mark a reef or shoal which is miles from the nearest port.

In the cardinal system the buoys show where a danger to navigation lies in relation to the mark. Buoys are placed in one or more of the four quadrants around the danger based on the cardinal points of the compass, i.e. N, S, E, and W. Thus a north cardinal mark is placed in the quadrant north of the danger and this shows that there is deep water to the north of the buoy. This system has great merit when used off rocky coastlines because the buoys show the direction of safe water without the need for a chart. On the other hand, the system has severe limitations when used to mark narrow, winding channels, where the lateral system is much better.

IALA maritime buoyage system

In the early 1970s there were a series of groundings and collisions in the English Channel which could be directly linked to the confusion caused by the different national buoyage systems, and fifty-seven seamen were drowned.

These tragedies galvanised the maritime nations into action, and in 1973 the International Association of Lighthouse Authorities (IALA) tried to find a new buoyage system which could be used world-wide. They came up with a proposal that was acceptable to most countries, and in 1980 everybody agreed to the basic concept. Under the IALA Maritime Buoyage System, as it is called, the world is divided into two regions. All Commonwealth countries (except Canada) are in Region A. Region B includes the USA and Japan. Here there are slight changes to some of the marks.

The changeover to the new system has been completed in Australia and New Zealand, and in most other countries.

The IALA system uses the best features of the two older systems and five types of marks are used:

1. *Lateral:* indicates the port and starboard sides of a channel.
2. *Cardinal:* indicates on which side of a mark the safe water lies.
3. *Isolated danger:* The mark is built or moored over a rock or a shoal of limited extent.
4. *Safe water:* shows there is deep water on each side of the mark. These marks may be used as mid-channel or landfall buoys.
5. *Special marks:* show such things as spoil ground, telegraph cables, pipelines or sewer outfalls. The chart must usually be consulted to find the purpose of a special mark.

Colours and lights

The colours red and green are reserved for port and starboard buoys and lights. Special marks are yellow with yellow lights. Other navigation marks show a white light and are distinguished from each other by the characteristics rigidly laid down and given below.

Topmarks

These are the most important feature in the daytime recognition of the function of an IALA mark. The only topmarks used are can, conical, spherical, and X-shaped.

Lateral marks

Port hand buoys mark the port or left hand side of a channel when going into harbour. They are red and can-shaped with an optional red can topmark, showing a red light of any characteristic by night. Beacons and spar or pillar buoys are painted red with a red can topmark, showing a red light.

Starboard hand buoys mark the starboard or right hand side of a channel when going into harbour. They are green and conical-shaped with an optional green cone topmark (point up). Beacons and spar or pillar buoys are painted green with a green cone topmark. Lights on buoys or beacons are green, and may have any characteristic.

When leaving harbour the buoys are reversed, i.e. to stay in the channel the red can buoys must be on the starboard side of the boat and the green conical buoys on the port side.

If port and/or starboard buoys are used in other than harbour areas, they are laid in accordance with what is called the general direction of buoyage, and this follows a clockwise direction around the coast. Where there could be any confusion, the general direction is indicated on the chart by the symbol shown below, which is magenta in colour. In this example a boat should leave red buoys to port, and green buoys to starboard when going in a counter-clockwise direction.

Preferred channel buoys or beacons can be used where a channel divides into two. Inevitably one of the channels will be deeper or wider than the other, and the red or green lateral marks can be modified to show which is the deeper or preferred channel. A lateral mark will be placed at the point where the channel divides. If the main channel is to the right, it will be a red port hand mark, but will have a green horizontal stripe around it. So if treated as a port hand mark, a boat will go to the right up the deep channel. But if looked on as a starboard hand mark due to the green stripe, a boat could go to the left, into the perfectly safe but shallower secondary channel.

Where the main channel is to the left, a green starboard hand mark is laid, but it has a red horizontal stripe to show that there are two channels. If any lights are fitted, they will show the main channel by being either red or green to match the main colour of the buoy. To indicate that there are two channels, the light characteristics will be composite group flashing, i.e., Fl (2 + 1). In practical terms this means that the lights will flash twice, pause, flash once, and then keep repeating this cycle.

GENERAL
DIRECTION OF
BUOYAGE ON
THIS CHART

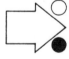

Fig. 34 *IALA chart symbol*

Cardinal marks

Cardinal marks are placed in one or more of the four quadrants around a navigation danger. (See diagrams at front and back inside covers of this book.) Individual marks take their names from the quadrant in which they are placed. Safe water lies to the north of an N mark, to the east of an E mark and so on. They are all pillar or spar buoys, painted in black and yellow horizontal bands and fitted with black double cone topmarks which will be the most important distinguishing feature by day. On a north buoy the cones are point up and on a south buoy, point down. The topmark on a west buoy is *w*asp-*w*aisted (W). In contrast, the east buoy is most decidedly *e*gg-shaped (E).

The points of the cones give the clue to the black band or bands, i.e.:

N	points up	Black band over yellow band
S	points down	Black band below yellow band
E	points outward	Black band above and below yellow band
W	points inward	Black band between upper and lower yellow band

At night cardinal marks are distinguished by showing white lights and the characteristics indicate the quadrant.

North mark	Quick flashing or very quick flashing
East mark	Groups of 3 quick or very quick flashes
South mark	Groups of 6 quick or very quick flashes followed by a long flash
West mark	Groups of 9 quick or very quick flashes

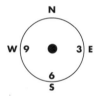

The number of flashes in each quadrant can be remembered by comparing them with the hours on a clock face, i.e., 3 h: E, 6 h: S, 9 h: W. The long flash after each group of 6 flashes on a south mark is to prevent it from being mistaken for a group of either 3 or 9 flashes. If two north marks are placed close together, one will be Q and the other VQ to avoid confusion between the two.

The following list shows some typical light descriptions for cardinal marks:

North mark	VQ or Q
East mark	VQ(3) 5 s
South mark	Q(6) + LFl 10 s
West mark	Q(9) 15 s

Isolated danger marks

Isolated danger marks are coloured black, with one or more red horizontal bands. Moored marks are spar or pillar buoys passable on either side. The main distinguishing feature by day is a black double sphere topmark and by night a white Fl(2) light. *Note:* Remember — two spheres, two flashes.

41

Safe water marks

Safe water marks have red and white vertical stripes and moored buoys may be pillar, spar or spherical. The pillar and spar should be fitted with a single red sphere topmark and by night lighted safe water marks will show an occulting, isophase or single long flash white light.

Special marks

All special marks are yellow with an optional single yellow X topmark. Any light carried will be yellow with a characteristic which cannot be mistaken for those used for the white lights of cardinal, isolated danger or safe water marks. In all probability the light will be flashing yellow.

Apart from the uses given earlier, special marks may be used to show a channel within a channel. For example, where the limits of a wide channel are already marked by red and green lateral buoys but only part of the width is suitable for deep draught vessels, the boundaries of the deep channel may be indicated by yellow buoys of the correct lateral shape, i.e., can or conical. The yachtsman should understand that channels marked by special buoys are reserved for deep draught vessels only, and if he is foolish enough to enter one at the same time as a supertanker, steam will *not* give way to sail!

The working of the IALA system is illustrated on the inside covers. The harbour is entered by passing between the red can and green conical buoys marking the headlands. The system is flexible and cardinal marks can be used in conjunction with lateral marks. The seaward end of the shoal could have been marked with a preferred channel buoy (red can with green stripe), but the harbour authorities have used a cardinal mark instead. This west cardinal buoy would be directly ahead and a vessel can pass the shoal safely by going between either of the two pairs of port and starboard hand buoys. At night the red lighted buoys are left to port, and the green lighted buoys to starboard when entering the harbour. A vessel would automatically go up the main channel after dark because the red and green buoys in the other do not have any lights.

Other IALA marks shown are the black and red isolated danger buoy over rough rock, and the south cardinal buoy to keep vessels clear of a wreck.

The general direction of the buoyage symbol shows that, on a coastal passage, port and starboard lateral marks are obeyed if the vessel is proceeding in an easterly direction. Of course when leaving harbour or going the opposite way to the general direction symbol, green buoys are left to port and red buoys to starboard.

Chapter Four
The Magnetic Compass

A compass is an instrument that indicates direction. Large vessels have gyroscopic compasses that show true directions. These true compasses are available for fitting in larger yachts, but at prices beyond the means of most people. Most small boats use a magnetic compass, which is one of the oldest of the navigator's instruments. Despite the popular theory that magnetic lodestone was adapted by the Chinese more than a thousand years ago to form a crude compass, the identity of the original 'inventors' is in doubt.

The magnetism in any bar magnet is concentrated near each end, called the poles of the magnet. The earth is a magnet and its poles are near, but not at, the true north and south poles. The earth's magnetic field consists of lines of magnetic force joining the north and south magnetic poles. A magnet hung on a piece of thread by its centre point or pivoted so that it is free to turn horizontally will line up in the earth's field with the same end always pointing towards the north magnetic pole. You can prove this by using an ordinary darning needle — most of them are magnetised — sticking it through a piece of straw floated in a bowl of water and slowly rotating the bowl. (In fact, the very first magnetic compasses consisted of a needle, a piece of straw and a bowl of water.) Note that the needle stays pointing in the same fixed direction, i.e., magnetic north. In practice this means that when altering course a boat turns around the magnet in the compass, although it may look as if the compass card is turning as the numbers flash past. The reader who understands this point will have less trouble in understanding other points about the magnetic compass.

If a compass rose was attached to a single bar magnet with its 0°–180° line along the length of the magnet, the rose would be kept aligned to magnetic north, no matter which way the boat turned. Any given direction could be read off the rose or *compass card* as it is then called. In a modern compass, the single magnet is replaced by a number of short, thin magnets parallel to each other which increase the directive power. These in turn are attached to the compass card in line with or parallel to the north-south axis. The card is pivoted on a jewelled bearing in a non-magnetic metal bowl with a glass top. While this would be acceptable on land, the movement in a boat would cause the card to swing to and fro around north. In trying to follow this movement, the helmsman would steer a zigzag instead of a steady course. The bowl is filled with liquid, commonly 45 per cent alcohol and 55 per cent water. Part of the weight of the card is taken by the buoyancy of the liquid, thus absorbing boat vibration and damping out the unwanted oscillations. There may also be a small air chamber in the centre of the card that further reduces the weight on the pivot, giving it a longer life. The alcohol lowers the freezing point of the liquid so that it doesn't ice up in very low temperatures.

The *lubber line* is the name given to a mark etched on the compass bowl which represents the bow or centre line of the boat. Thus to steer any given course, the boat is turned until the lubber line has been brought directly opposite the correct heading on the compass card. Think about that. The card stays still. The lubber line goes where the bow goes. It follows that an error in steering will be introduced if the lubber line is not exactly parallel to the centre or keel line of the boat.

Steering compasses
Virtually all marine compasses are liquid filled, but three main varieties are used as steering compasses. In the traditional model the compass bowl has a circular glass plate cover. The internal magnets and compass card react to the horizontal component of the earth's magnetic field and the card may stick if the bowl is stood on its side, for example, when the boat rolls, so the whole compass may be mounted in gimbals. The *Concise*

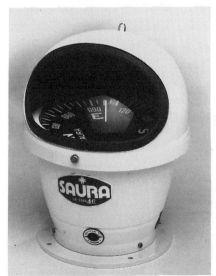

Fig. 35 *Dome type steering compass*

Fig. 36 *Grid steering compass*

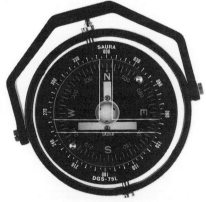

Oxford Dictionary defines these as being 'contrivances (usu. of rings and pivots) for keeping articles (esp. compass and chronometer) horizontal at sea', which sums them up pretty well.

Compass cards are generally marked in the circular 0°–360° notation and the course is read off against a lubber line on the forward side of the bowl. If all 360 degrees were shown on the card of a small boat's compass, the graduations would be difficult to read. Some makers overcome this problem by only marking the card every five degrees with bolder graduations. The figures are also made larger and more distinct by leaving out the last numeral, e.g., 4 is 40°, 10 is 100°, 24 is 240°, and so on. Others fit the compass with a magnifier that enlarges the lubber line and the graduations immediately either side of it. Many compasses are fitted with a clear dome, which itself magnifies the card, and are internally gimballed. The compass is fixed to the superstructure and rolls with the boat, but the card and lubber line are attached to a cage that can tilt inside the bowl, remaining level at all times. The third variety, called a grid steering compass, is described shortly.

In order to steer an accurate course when using a lubber line fitted compass, the instrument must be directly in front of the helmsman. If he is to one side or the other of the compass, the change in perspective leads to a false impression of exactly which graduation is opposite the lubber line. This slight error in course due to the apparent change in position of the lubber line, caused by a change in the observer's position, is called *parallax*.

In boats where the helmsman has no choice as to position, one way around the problem is to put the craft on the correct heading with the eye directly behind the compass, then move quickly to the steering

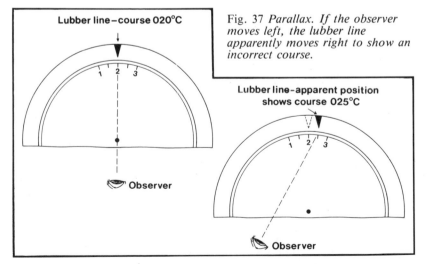

Fig. 37 *Parallax. If the observer moves left, the lubber line apparently moves right to show an incorrect course.*

position, read off the apparent course and steer it. Naturally if the helmsman is forced to change position for any reason, the apparent course must be reassessed.

Grid steering compass

Attempting to steer a steady course over a long period when using the conventional lubber line compass can cause eye strain, and there is always the parallax problem. On the other hand, the human eye is able to tell when two lines are exactly parallel to each other and can detect the slight difference of alignment between them if they shift even marginally out of parallel. This property is utilised in the grid steering compass, where the helmsman can hold a course to an accuracy of about one degree by steering the boat so as to keep two lines parallel.

The compass card in these instruments may or may not have degrees marked on it, but it will have a line or arrow marking the north-south (0°–180°) axis of the card. A rotatable glass plate cover fits over the fixed glass cover on the compass bowl, and has two parallel lines, the outline of a solid arrow or a T-shape engraved or painted on it as in Fig. 36. This is the *grid*. The rotatable cover is graduated from 0° – 360° and the grid lines or arrow are oriented along its 0° – 180° axis. The compass bowl will, as usual, have a fixed lubber line indicating the bow of the boat.

The principle of operation is a bit difficult to grasp at first, but well worth the effort. To steer a given course, such as north, the glass cover is rotated until its 0° is opposite the lubber line on the compass bowl and then clamped in position. The boat is turned to a northerly heading by altering course until the grid lines are either side of and parallel to the north-south line on the compass card. Course is maintained by keeping these lines parallel. Where there is a T-shape, the head of the T can be used if the helmsman is out to the side of the compass. To alter course to, say, east, the cover plate is rotated until the 090° graduations on it are opposite the lubber line, as in Fig. 39. The boat is again turned until the grid lines are parallel to the north-south line on the compass card — at this time the boat will be heading 090°.

To steer any given course, the steps are:

1. Turn the rotatable plate until the required heading is opposite the lubber line and clamp it in position.

2. Alter course until grid and compass lines are parallel and steer the boat to keep them that way.

The grid compass is most useful with the boat on a steady course during a coastal or ocean passage. It has some limitations when frequent alterations of course would call for continual resetting of the grid. Examples are when a yacht is being sailed hard on the wind or any boat is passing through a winding but unmarked channel, and the navigator should keep an accurate track by maintaining steady headings on each

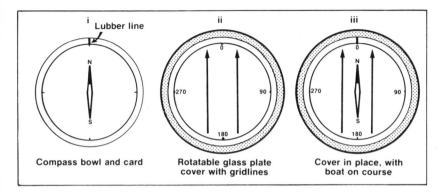

i Lubber line

ii

iii

Compass bowl and card

Rotatable glass plate
cover with gridlines

Cover in place, with
boat on course

Fig. 38 (i) *Compass bowl and card* (ii) *Rotatable glass plate cover with gridlines* (iii) *Cover in place, with boat on course 000°C*

leg. The instrument is essentially a steering compass because, to give the helmsman a clear view of the grid lines, it may have to be sited rather lower than a conventional lubber line compass. Even if it is fitted high enough to give an all-round view and thus be fitted with a sighting device, it could not be used for taking bearings unless the card were marked in degrees as well as the north-south line or arrow.

Cost
Good steering compasses are expensive but worth the money. The cheaper

Fig. 39 *Altering course* (i) *The boat is on a northerly heading, but the grid cover is set for course 090°* (ii) *Halfway through the turn* (iii) *When the lines are again parallel, the boat is on the new course*

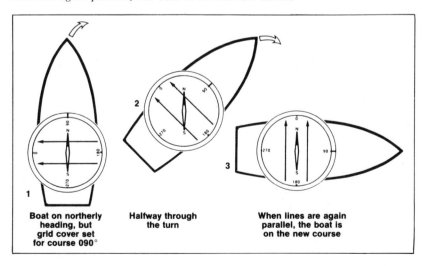

1 Boat on northerly
heading, but
grid cover set
for course 090°

Halfway through
the turn

When lines are again
parallel, the boat is
on the new course

47

models from reputable manufacturers are also reliable, but they may need more frequent checking for errors, especially after the boat has been through a season or so of rough weather, than their more durable and larger relatives. The rule of thumb for those intending to take to the high seas is to decide what you can afford, double it and then go out and buy one at twice the price. It is wise to look on those advertisements offering 'amazing value' with genuine amazement.

The fluxgate compass

The solid-state fluxgate compass is an electronic hybrid which is halfway between the traditional magnetic compass, and the expensive gyro-based systems. It has no magnet as such but still relies on the earth's magnetic field for its directive force. The big advantage is that it can drive up to four repeating compasses in other parts of the boat. Magnetic variation can be set on the equipment, which then gives true directions.

The heart of the fluxgate compass is a specially wound coil called a toroid which creates a uniform magnetic field around itself. A secondary coil is wound on the toroid. While the toroid's magnetic field remains uniform no voltage is induced in the secondary coil. But the toroid is extremely sensitive and when the external lines of force of the earth's magnetic field act on it the toroid's magnetic field changes. This change induces a voltage in the secondary winding. The size of the voltage is proportional to the angle at which the toroid, and therefore the boat, cuts the earth's magnetic lines of force and is a measure of heading, or change of heading. This voltage is fed to a repeater, which shows the boat's magnetic course.

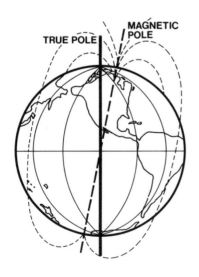

Fig. 40 *North magnetic pole*

The earth's field or magnetic flux can be distorted by boat magnetism, so the fluxgate electronic sensor is subject to deviation like any ordinary compass. This can be corrected by a compass adjuster or using a deviation card to apply a correction. But as one of the repeating compasses can be installed at the steering position, the sensor can be sited in the position where there is least magnetic interference.

The north magnetic pole

Any magnetic compass that indicates the exact direction of magnetic north is working perfectly. However, it does not show true direction because the true and magnetic north poles are over 700 miles apart. The fact that a magnetic compass does not show true directions is annoying, but no fault of the instrument.

Seafarers knew from early times that their compasses did not show true north, but practical interest in the location of the north magnetic pole in the form of an organised search for it did not take place until 1818 with the Royal Navy's campaign to discover the North-West Passage. It was found by James Ross in 1831 on the west side of the Boothia peninsula in the Canadian north-west territories. Ross was also the first man to reach the south magnetic pole some ten years later. He was able to detect that the north magnetic pole was moving, but he could not predict the movement with his limited instruments and in the time available to him.

In 1990 the pole was at 81° north, 109° west which is north-west of King Christian Island, and it is moving across the Canadian arctic at about 15 miles a year.

Variation

The angle or difference in degrees between the direction of magnetic north and true north at any place is called *variation*. If magnetic north lies to the right or east of true north the variation is said to be easterly, and if to the left, westerly.

Variation differs from place to place on the earth's surface. As the magnetic poles are moving slowly, the variation at any place changes slightly from year to year. The value of variation for a particular year and the annual change in minutes are shown on the inner or magnetic ring of coastal charts in one of two ways. In Fig. 41 the variation for 1984 is 19° 06′E, increasing 4′ annually. Variation in 1994 would be 19° 46′E or 20°E for practical purposes.

The navigator will find that many charts use this method for some years to come. However, in new editions of often-used charts the IHO method of giving variation will be shown. Look at Fig. 41a. Here the value, year and change in variation are combined in one caption along the magnetic north arrow. So 19° 20′ E 1994 (2′ E) means that the annual easterly increase is 2 minutes. With an easterly variation, 1994 (2′ W)

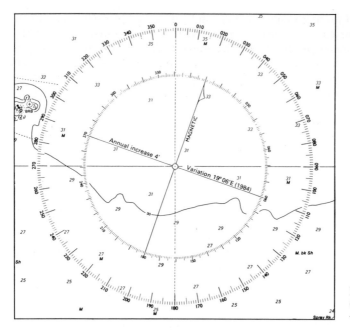

Fig. 41 and 41a
Compass rose
— variation

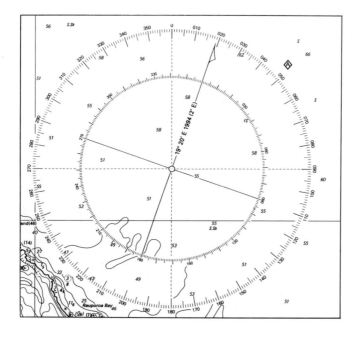

means that the variation is effectively moving west, or decreasing 2 minutes each year.

Directions in chartwork are primarily based on true north. Magnetic directions are given the suffix M to distinguish them from true directions, e.g., magnetic north and east are written as 000°M and 090°M. The reader should make it a habit to write any magnetic direction in this way, because Murphy's Rule applies — if it is not done, any confusion about which is which will occur at the worst possible time.

Magnetic directions could be measured directly from the magnetic ring. There can be three problems here. First, the graduations are smaller than those on the outer ring and more difficult to read. Second, the alignment is fully correct only in the year for which the variation is given. Lastly, there is no magnetic ring on many international charts.

A line on a chart joining all points that have the same variation for a given time is called a magnetic variation curve or isogonal. The isogonals — for each whole degree change of variation — are printed on the charts as shown in Fig. 4?. The actual variation is printed somewhere along each curve, together with the annual change in minutes, and using the E/W convention described above. The year is given in the title.

Fig. 42 *Curves of magnetic variation*

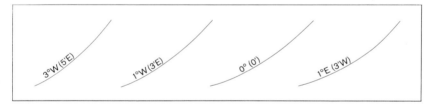

Conversion

The initial problem is to convert a true course taken from the chart to a magnetic course to steer. The various texts give several ways of remembering how to do this. I believe that the ultimate test of a rule or method is that it works in a howling gale when the chart table is awash, the skipper is screaming for the course to steer and the navigator is about to throw up. In such circumstances drawing diagrams is out, and so is trying to visualise the problem. The less thinking required the better.

Look at Fig. 43; true N and E are shown. The variation is 10°E, which means that magnetic north is 10° to the right of true north. 000°M is the same direction as 010°T, 090°M is equivalent to 100°T. In each case the magnetic reading is 10° less than the true for the same direction. A rhyme for remembering how to convert a true course to magnetic goes:
Variation east, magnetic least,
Variation west, magnetic best, e.g.:

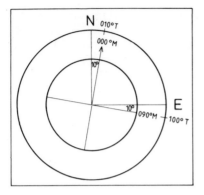

Fig. 43 *Variation is 10°E*

True course	100°T	010°T	064°T
Variation east	− 10°E	− 10°E	− 10°E
Magnetic course (least)	090°M	000°M	054°M

A westerly variation is added to give a magnetic course which is best, or greater than the true, e.g.:

True course	100°T	180°T	236°T
Variation west	+ 10°W	+ 6°W	+ 12°W
Magnetic course	110°M	186°M	248°M

Magnetic to true

The above rhyme still applies in that a magnetic course containing easterly variation is least, i.e., less than the equivalent true course. Therefore the variation must be added, e.g.:

Magnetic course (least)	047°M	333°M	291°M
Variation east	+ 10°E	+ 2°E	+ 14°E
True course	057°T	335°T	305°T

With westerly variation, the magnetic direction is best or the greater of the two so it must be subtracted to find the true:

Magnetic course (best)	037°M	213°M	347°M
Variation west	− 10°W	- 4°W	− 16°W
True course	027°T	209°T	331°T

Many navigators will spend most of their boating life in the one general area and may have to contend only with the one type of variation. Due to the slow annual change, the value may only vary a few degrees during their lifetime. For these folk, the conversion of true to magnetic and vice versa will become automatic with a little practice. Nevertheless, although the navigator can quieten a screaming skipper by doing a quick mental sum, it always pay to check the answer afterwards with a pencil and paper.

In summary, the principle of finding direction using a magnetic compass is to pivot a compass card in a non-magnetic, liquid-filled bowl to dampen the shocks, and let the magnets line up in the earth's field. Then, allowing for a known variation, any true direction can be found or steered. So what happens? The instrument is mounted in a boat. If it is a steel or ferro-cement craft the hull or metal in it will almost certainly be slightly magnetised. An engine with a magnetic field of its own will be installed underneath or near it. The compass may be near a tachometer in the instrument panel. The new VHF or SSB set is installed nearby because that is the only place left for it. The magnetic fields in these are very strong indeed. Then the helmsman may drape a transistor radio over it to while away the long night hours. For good measure a magnetic torch is put on the nearest piece of metal to the compass so that it is nice and handy. Finally, the spare metal tools are bundled into the locker underneath it.

It seems that we take every possible step not only to shield the compass from the earth's field so that it can't line up but then to actively throw in other fields. Each one of these will tend to deflect the compass card away from magnetic north, but luckily for us some of these stray fields will neutralise each other. Even so, someone may say in utter disbelief, 'There is something wrong with this compass — it's a few degrees out!'

The 'few degrees out', due to the combined effects of every piece of magnetised metal in the boat's hull and objects near the compass, is called *deviation*. It is an error.

Deviation

Deviation is the angular deflection of the compass card away from magnetic north, i.e., the difference in degrees between the direction of magnetic north and the direction the compass indicates as being north. If the compass settles to the right of magnetic north, the deviation is easterly and, if to the left, westerly. Directions by compass are given the suffix C to distinguish them from true or magnetic directions. For example, compass north is written as 000°C.

Whereas variation is the same for every boat in the same general area, deviation differs from boat to boat. It may also vary in different parts of the same boat. The deviation in a compass is not constant; it changes with and is dependent on the boat's course or heading. Briefly, this is because a vessel crosses or cuts the earth's magnetic lines of force at different angles, depending on heading. Some of the magnetism in the boat's hull varies according to this angle of cut with the earth's field. However, for any given course all the directions as indicated by a compass will be in error by the amount of deviation on that course. The reasons for the changing deviations can be seen from Fig. 44. Any magnetised metal having a deviating effect changes position in relation to the compass needle as the boat is turned around the compass card. Remember that

53

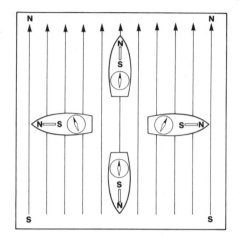

Fig. 44 *Changing deviations*

the latter attempts to stay pointing in the one fixed direction, i.e., magnetic north. In Fig. 44, a magnet is forward of and in line with the compass with its south end towards the compass needle.

If the boat is on either a north or south magnetic heading, the magnet is acting along the length of the compass needle and in line with the earth's magnetic field and there is no deviating effect. If the boat is heading east, there is a different situation. The magnet is acting across the earth's magnetic lines of force. The south end of the magnet attracts the north end of the compass needle and repels its south end. The needle pivots clockwise, giving an easterly deviation. If the boat is on a westerly heading, the situation is reversed and a westerly deviation is induced. This is an oversimplification in that other magnetised metal may induce deviation with the boat on a north-south heading and none on an east or west course. The final deviation in each heading is a combination of the various forces acting on the compass needle, each of which changes its position in relation to the compass card as the boat is turned onto the various headings.

Deviation card

The process of compensating for excess deviation is called *compass adjustment* and is best left to a professional compass adjuster. However, in a small boat, if the deviations do not exceed about 5° they are determined for the various headings and allowed for in the same way as variation. The process of finding the deviations is called *swinging the compass*. It can be done by the amateur and is explained in the next chapter. The deviations are recorded on a card which should be mounted over the chart table for easy reference. Ideally the deviation should be known every 20° starting at compass north, i.e., on 18 headings. In a small boat, eight headings will suffice — the cardinal points N, S, E and

W and the inter-cardinal points NE, SE, SW, and NW as shown on page 56.

The rhyme given earlier can be adapted for use in converting a compass course to a magnetic by changing two words:

Deviation east, *compass* least
Deviation west, *compass* best

For example, using the deviations in the Deviation Card, page 56:

Compass course	006°C	102°C	224°C	276°C
Deviation	− 4°W	− 2°W	+ 5°E	+ 2°E
Magnetic course	002°M	100°M	229°M	278°M

Once the magnetic course is known, the true course can be found by applying variation; i.e., to convert 088°C to true using the Deviation Card and assuming the variation to be 10°E, the deviation for 090°C, which is the nearest course given in the table, is 3°W.

Compass course		088°C
Deviation	−	3°W
Magnetic course		085°M
Variation	+	10°E
True course		095°T

I repeat two points made earlier. Firstly, every reading on the compass in this example has an error of 3°W due to deviation. Secondly, the deviation changes when a boat alters course. Any bearings taken with the compass must never be used when finding deviation from the table; it must always be entered with the boat's heading at the time. So, with the boat on course 088°C for which the deviation is 3°W, if the bearings of two shore objects using this compass were found to be 180°C and 270°C, the true bearings would be:

Compass bearing	180°C	270°C
Deviation	− 3°W	− 3°W
Magnetic bearing	177°M	267°M
Variation	+ 10°E	+ 10°E
True bearing	187°T	277°T

True to compass

A more common problem is finding the compass course to steer for a true course taken from the chart. The working is done in the reverse order to that just outlined, e.g., to find the required compass course for a heading of 248°T, if the variation is 20°E:

True course	248°T
Variation	− 20°E
Magnetic course (least)	228°M

Deviation Card		
Heading by compass		Deviation
N	000°	4° W
NE	045°	6° W
E	090°	3° W
SE	135°	1° E
S	180°	4° E
SW	225°	5° E
W	270°	2° E
NW	315°	1° W
N	360°	4° W

The deviation cannot be found until this part of the problem has been worked because it is dependent on heading by compass. 228°M is not the compass course either, unless there is no deviation on this heading. But, being the closest value we have at this stage, the magnetic course is used to enter the deviation table. From the Deviation Card, the nearest compass course is 225°C, so deviation is 5°E.

Magnetic course	228°M
Deviation	– 5°E
Compass course (least)	223°C

No time need be lost while doing the conversion if a large alteration of course is needed in a hurry. Simply tell the helmsman to steer the new true course by compass; i.e., if the required heading is 020°T, turn to 020°C. Assuming that variation is 10°E and deviation 4°W in this example, the final course would be 014°C. A further 6° adjustment brings the boat onto the required heading.

Deviation brings with it some side effects that may not be immediately apparent. If the boat runs into heavy rain or fog and the skipper decides to go back, the obvious thing to do is to reverse course. Ignoring for the moment the effect of current, which is discussed in Chapter Six, this cannot be done by merely turning 180° by compass. An example will show why not. Assume that the course is 000°C and the deviation is 4°E. The magnetic course is therefore 004°M. If the deviation on 180°C were 4°W, this heading would be 176°M. Thus, while turning 180° by compass, the actual turn would be 176°M – 004°M or 172°, and the vessel has not reversed course. That 8° error would at best confuse proceedings, at worst put the boat on the rocks.

If visibility is reducing after leaving harbour and there is no deviation table on board, the navigator should take the precaution of turning the boat to point at the harbour entrance or direction of safe return and read the compass heading. Then if the decision is later made to go back, course is reversed by steering the compass course found by experiment.

Chapter Five
Swinging the Compass

The bittacle is a square box nailed together with wooden pinnes, because iron nails would attract the Compasse.
John Smith, English soldier and adventurer, 1627

John Smith was talking about the modern-day binnacle, which is the wooden structure used to house large compasses. While he and his contemporaries knew of the existence of deviation, they did not understand how to correct for it, nor, indeed, how to find it.

There are now half a dozen or more procedures for finding deviation, but none is applicable to all types of boat. Five of the methods commonly used are described here, with notes on their limitations. The easiest and quickest is given first, but it can only be considered as a check because the errors may only be accurate to plus or minus one degree. However, the results will show if there are excess deviations in the steering compass, in which case a compass adjuster should be called in. As in all the methods, the boat must be well clear of the shoreline, wharves and jetties and any large metal objects that might induce random deviations, such as harbour buoys. It is not suitable for steel-hulled craft.

Compass comparison

A hand bearing compass is unlikely to have any error if used well aft away from the deviating forces in the boat's hull (see page 84). Thus deviation can be found by comparing the heading by steering compass and that by hand bearing compass. The boat is steadied on each of the eight cardinal and inter-cardinal headings in turn and the compass allowed to settle. The magnetic heading is found by taking a bearing of the bow with the hand compass from a centre line position. This is compared with the course by steering compass read off at the same time. Any difference between the two is the deviation on that heading, e.g.:

Magnetic heading (HBC)	040°M
Compass heading	− 038°C (least)
Deviation	2°E

The centre line position at the stern can be judged in two ways. The first is to mark the centres of the mast and the after end of the cabin roof. The navigator moves so that the two marks are seen to be in line and is then looking along the fore and aft line of the boat, i.e., directly towards the bow. A bearing of the centre of the mast gives the boat's magnetic course. A second method is to put sighting marks consisting of coloured tape on either side of the centre of the pulpit, so that when the navigator is sighting directly along the fore and aft line from the stern centre line position, the mast is exactly between the marks. Here again, a bearing of the centre of the mast gives the magnetic course.

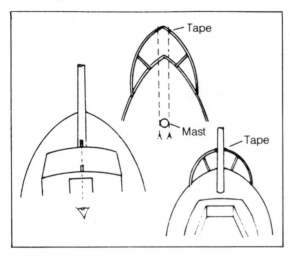

Fig. 45a, b and c
The use of tape or sighting marks in judging the centre line

Using a transit

If the steering compass has a clear all-round field of view and is fitted with a sighting device similar to that on a hand bearing compass, the use of a transit will give more accurate results. Choose two well-defined objects on the chart that can be brought into line with each other when seen from a boat in the harbour or off the coast. When in line, they are said to be *in transit*. The boat is run across the transit on the required headings and the bearing taken as the marks come into line. The difference between this figure and the magnetic bearing is the deviation. Two things are essential — calm sea conditions, and the boat must be held steady on course while crossing the transit.

Fig. 46 shows a suitable pair of marks. Their bearing when in line is 060°T. If the variation were 6° west, the magnetic bearing would be 066°M.

The results should be noted methodically, as shown on page 59. A deviation card could be made up using the information in the first and last columns.

Compass heading		Transit bearing	Compass bearing	Deviation
N	000°C	066°M	069°C	3°W
NE	045°C	066°M	070°C	4°W
E	090°C	066°M	067°C	1°W
SE	135°C	066°M	064°C	2°E
S	180°C	066°M	062°C	4°E
SW	225°C	066°M	063°C	3°E
W	270°C	066°M	065°C	1°E
NW	315°C	066°M	068°C	2°W
N	360°C	066°M	069°C	3°W

Bearing of a distant object

The position of the boat must be known and the bearing of a shore object taken from the chart. The deviations can be found with the boat at anchor or under way, but remaining within 100 metres of the known spot, which should be marked by a small buoy or float secured to the sea bed. If at anchor, the bow is put on the various headings by using a helper in a rowboat to tow the stern around. If the boat is under way, the bearing is taken as the boat passes close to the marker on each heading. The minimum range of the shore object should be 5 miles when at anchor and 10 miles if under way. The deviation on each heading is the difference between the bearing by compass and the magnetic bearing found from the chart.

The anchor method is suitable for yachts because, as when sailing, the engine is stopped. Power boats at anchor should have the engine running because this is the normal operating state. Yacht navigators should realise that the deviations may change with the auxiliary engine running. It may be necessary to have two deviation cards, one for use under sail and the other when under power.

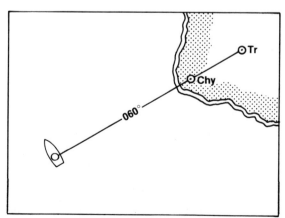

Fig. 46 *Running a transit to find deviation*

Unknown distant object

Deviation can be found by using a shore object even if the bearing is not known because the mark is uncharted or cannot be identified. Its magnetic bearing can be found by averaging the compass bearings taken on eight equally spaced courses. These bearings contain variation, which is constant in the one area, and deviation, which changes with heading. The assumption made is that the total easterly deviations are equal to the total westerly ones. In averaging the compass bearings, the deviations are therefore eliminated and the answer contains only variation, i.e., it is the magnetic bearing. The assumption is justified in a wooden yacht where the compass is mounted on the centre line or in a boat where there is an existing deviation card. If the totals of east and west deviations found previously are within 2° of each other, and there have been no major structural alterations or installations since the last swing, satisfactory results should be obtained. However, this method is not recommended for other craft.

The working can be illustrated by assuming that the bearing of the marks shown on page 59 was not known, but that the compass bearings had been taken. The eight headings were:

Headings by compass	Bearing
N	069° C
NE	070° C
E	067° C
SE	064° C
S	062° C
SW	063° C
W	065° C
NW	068° C

$$8\overline{)528°}$$
$$066°M$$

The average is the same as the magnetic bearing found using the chart.

Series of transits

Many boats have neither a sighting device nor a clear view from the steering compass in the cockpit or control position, and finding deviations is no five-minute job. It may take an hour or more. There are several ways of overcoming the problem, but the procedure given below requires the minimum of equipment. It is not suitable for a yacht under sail.

A series of transits is used, chosen so that the magnetic bearings conform as closely as possible to the cardinal and inter-cardinal headings. The boat is run along each transit in turn and the difference between the heading by compass and the magnetic bearing is the deviation on that heading.

The procedure is illustrated in Fig. 47. The navigator was not able to

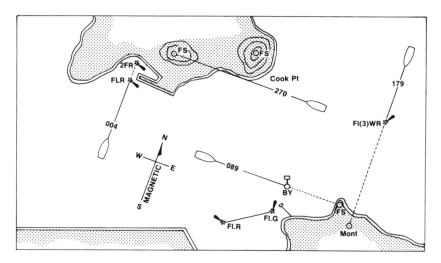

Fig. 47 *Running a series of transits*

find marks that would give magnetic N, E, S and W exactly, but the transits bearing 004°M, 089°M, 179°M and 268°M are close enough to give accurate deviations. The results obtained are given in Fig. 48, which for brevity shows only the deviations on the four main headings. Notice the mix of marks used to get the transits — beacon with beacon, beacon with steep headland, beacon with flagstaff and light beacon with monument.

Readers may have a pleasant surprise if they closely study their own chart. There is a better than even chance that most of the eight sets of transits needed can be found within a couple of miles of their moorings. The major problem is in boat handling. The chosen objects must not only be in line when each reading is taken, but the bow must be pointing at the marks as in Fig. 49a. In Fig. 49b the marks are not in line, even though the bow is aimed at the front mark. Fig 49c shows that the marks would be in line but the compass heading is not correct because the bow is off to port of the line of the transit. The procedure must be carried out in calm conditions with little or no crosstide.

Fig. 48 *The comparison between magnetic bearing of each transit and compass heading gives deviation*

Heading by compass	Transit bearing	Compass course	Deviation
N	004°M	007°C	3°W
E	089°M	090°C	1°W
S	179°M	175°C	4°E
W	268°M	267°C	1°E

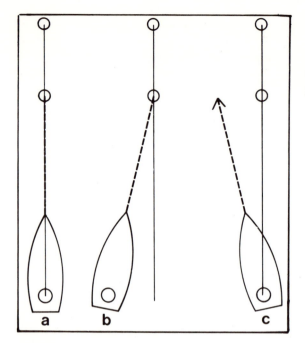

Fig. 49a, b and c
*Boat handling
problems when
running a transit*

a   b   c

Using a graph

Although the compass swing may have been done on only eight headings,
the deviation on any compass course can be found by drawing up a graph
of deviations obtained against headings by compass. Look at Fig. 50,
which shows the eight deviations listed on page 59. A smooth curve has
been drawn through these points. The deviation on a heading of 155°C,
for example, is found by laying a rule horizontally through this course
to find where it meets the curve, then vertically from this point to read
off the deviation as 3°E.

It was stated earlier that the transits used did not have to be exactly
magnetic north, east, etc. If the deviations obtained are plotted in this
visual form, the deviations on the cardinal and inter-cardinal headings
can be read off the graph when making up the deviation card.

Lubber line error

A compass course is read off against the lubber line which is the datum
mark for steering. The compass must be so mounted that a line joining
its pivot with the lubber line is parallel to the keel line of the boat. If
it is offset in any way, lubber line error is introduced. It is not due to
magnetic influences and is constant on all headings.

Fig. 51a shows a compass that has no error from this cause, nor any
deviation on the heading 069°C. Moving the lubber line will not put a
deviation in the compass card, but by physically turning the compass

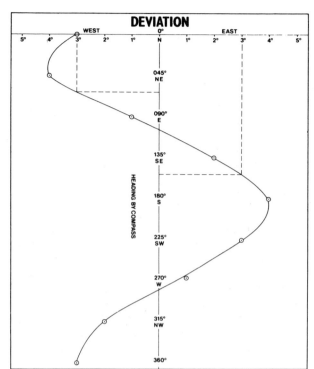

Fig. 50
Deviation curve

bowl 3° to starboard the course would read 072°C, as shown in Fig. 51b. The compass now has a 3° west lubber line error. However, notice that, regardless of the displacement of the line, the compass card has not moved and the direction in which the bow is pointing remains 069°C.

A point of confusion can arise when using a compass fitted with a sighting device that has a lubber line error. The error must be allowed

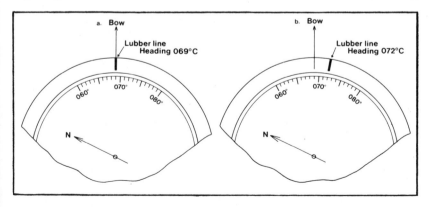

Fig. 51a and b *Lubber line error*

for when deciding courses to steer, but ignored when taking bearings using the sighting device. The answer, of course, is to get rid of the root cause by ensuring that the compass is set up correctly, as explained on page 68. If the error is found to exist, it is removed as follows:

If error is east, slew compass same number of degrees to starboard. If error is west, slew compass to port.

Checking results

A check can usually be made on the accuracy of the results obtained, but the checks vary depending on the particular method that was used to find the deviations.

Known bearing of a single transit or distant object
Add the compass bearings and divide by the number of headings, i.e., eight. The result should be within one degree of the magnetic bearing of the transit or mark. A difference of two or more degrees would indicate that one or more of the deviations found was inaccurate. This check cannot be done when an unknown distant object is used, because the magnetic bearing is found by averaging the eight bearings, and doing the same thing again would prove nothing. If the check proves satisfactory, lubber line error can be detected by running a single transit on any one of the eight headings. Compare the course by compass with the magnetic bearing of the transit. The difference is the error on that heading and it should be the same as the deviation already noted for that course. Any difference between the two is due to lubber line error, e.g., if the deviation found during the swing was 2°E and that found by running a transit on the same heading was 4°E, there would be a 2°E lubber line error in the compass.

Series of transits and comparisons with hand bearing compass
The errors found when using these methods include any lubber line error. This can be detected by adding the deviations on the headings N, S, E and W, calling east deviations plus and west deviations minus. In theory the sum should be zero; in practice it may be one or two degrees, which is acceptable. If it is greater, divide the total by four and the result is the number of degrees the lubber line is in error.

For example, the errors listed below contain a lubber line error of 3°W. Summing the deviations and dividing by four shows this:

```
N      − 7°W
E      − 5°W
S      + 1°E
W      − 1°W
    4 )12°W
        3°W lubber line error
```

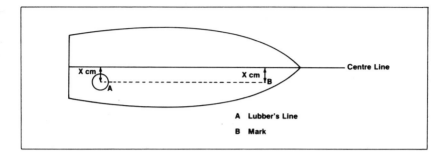

Fig. 52 *Checking the accuracy of a lubber line*

Once the compass is slewed and the error removed, the deviation card must be corrected, i.e., in the example above, the deviations would become:

N	4° W
E	2° W
S	4° E
W	2° E

Harbour tests

The accuracy of the results obtained using any of the methods for finding deviation depends largely on thorough preparation. One vital point is to check for lubber line error. In a centrally mounted compass a sighting across the centre line of the compass and the lubber line should lead directly across the bow or to the middle of the mast. If the steering compass is offset to one side, the distance between the compass centre and the fore and aft line of the boat must be measured. Place a mark as far forward as possible the same distance off centre. Now a sighting across the compass through the lubber line should pass through this mark, as in Fig. 52.

All magnetic materials should be moved well away from the compass. Electrical equipment in the vicinity, such as depth finder, windscreen wipers, refrigerator, radar set and instrument panel lighting should be switched on in turn and any effect on the compass card noted. It may be too late to resite any of these, but in any circumstances when steering a given course is critical to the safety of the boat, the navigator may be faced with a difficult decision. The choice may be between having cold beer or an accurate compass.

The card should be checked for friction by bringing a small magnet slowly towards the compass until the card is deflected 20° to 30°. When the card is steady, move the magnet quickly away. The card should move steadily back to within a degree or so of the original heading. A faulty pivot would cause the card to stick and repairs would be necessary.

65

Although a liquid compass should not have a bubble, it will operate satisfactorily provided that any bubble is less than 1/6 the diameter of the card. This will not satisfy the navigation theorist or the examiner. The textbooks state that any bubbles should be removed by turning the compass bowl upside down, allowing the air to work its way up through the liquid and then topping up through the filling plug with the mixture recommended by the manufacturer.

If the compass is the internally gimballed dome type, it should be rolled gently from side to side to simulate the rolling and pitching motion of a boat — the gimbals should be seen to be free and not sticking. However, bear in mind that many modern power boat compasses are only gimballed to compensate for a rolling motion and not for pitching.

The steering wheel should be turned slowly from amidships to hard over both sides, and the throttle and gear lever moved through their full working range. These movements should not alter the compass heading or make it swing. If they do, the compass will have to be resited. The engine should be started and any effects on the compass noted. In practice the card may kick as the engine starts, but there is no problem if it settles back to the original reading. The boat must be kept on a steady heading in calm conditions during this and all other harbour tests.

Compass checks

Deviation should be fully checked once a year, after a long lie-up in or out of the water, after major structural alterations or installations such as a new engine, and of course if a new compass is fitted. The navigator should try to check the deviation on at least one heading each time the boat goes to sea. If the result is within one degree or so of the value listed on the deviation card, it is reasonable to assume that none of the deviations has changed. If there is a marked difference, the whole card is suspect. The investigation should continue there and then, even if it consists only of a comparison against a hand bearing compass on the four cardinal headings. If the deviation has changed on two or more of these headings, a full compass swing should be carried out as soon as possible.

Remember that in fair weather cruising all the marks and coastal features can be clearly seen. When visibility is suddenly reduced by rain or fog, the humble compass rises sharply in status.

Heeling error

Certain of the magnetic influences in a boat act vertically through the compass. These are always present, but when the vessel is upright as in Fig. 53, no deviation is induced because the only effect is to try to tilt the needle on its pivot. This is overcome by pivoting the compass card well above its centre of gravity and the weight of the card keeps it horizontal. Also notice that most of the boat's hull is below the compass

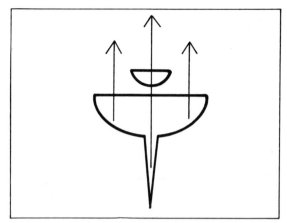

Fig. 53 *Upright vessel*

bowl. However, when a boat rolls, these forces may cause a deviation called *heeling error*.

When a vessel heels over, the compass in its gimbals remains horizontal. One side of the hull changes position in relation to the compass in that it moves from below to be in line with or even partly above the compass card. The latter is attracted to or deflected away from the high side, and as this alternates with each roll, the card takes on a swing which makes steering difficult. In a craft with a permanent list or a yacht heeled over in the wind, a steady deviation is introduced.

Although heeling error is directly related to the angle of heel, the deviation it causes for a given angle depends on the heading of the vessel. The maximum deviation is on a north or south magnetic course while it is virtually nil on east or west. The reason for this is shown in Fig. 55. With the bow headed north the compass needle is turned alternately from side to side as the vessel rolls. When headed east the heeling error effect is along the length of the needle and there is no deviating force.

If the navigator notices that the compass is oscillating badly in rough weather with the boat on a north-south heading, the cause is almost certainly heeling error. It may be tested for in a yacht by turning onto north or south by compass with the sheet eased, and heeling her over

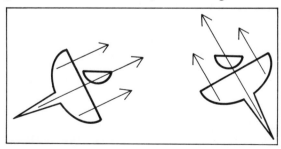

Fig. 54 *When a vessel heels the vertical forces acting on the compass acquire a horizontal component and introduce heeling error*

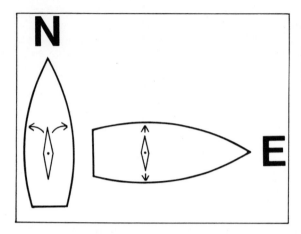

Fig. 55 *Heeling error*
a *On magnetic north*
b *East*

by hauling the sheet home. If the compass course alters radically, the error exists. The advice of a compass adjuster should be sought. He can test for and eliminate the deviating force in harbour using a crafty little gadget called, oddly enough, a heeling error instrument.

Installing a compass

When installing a compass, there are two requirements that often conflict. The first is that the card should be in plain view of the helmsman, whether he is sitting to windward or to leeward on either tack in a yacht. The second is that the compass should be sited in a magnetically neutral position. With the amount of electronic gear in a boat these days, this might sound like wishful thinking. However, the deviating force from any source decreases very quickly with a small increase in its distance from the compass. More correctly, it varies inversely as the square of the distance. For example, if there is 8° deviation from a source at 16 cm, by doubling the distance from the compass to 32 cm the deviation decreases to 2°.

Safe distances from the compass are laid down for the more common items of equipment but these vary from 1 m to 2.5 m and may not be obtainable in many boats. In the following guide, the distances should be considered an absolute minimum. For engine instruments and tachometers, steel steering shafts and gearing, windscreen wiper motors, throttles and gear shifts this minimum distance is 30 cm. With depth finders, radio speakers, microphones and other items with internal magnets the distance should be no less than 60 cm. For the engine, steel exhaust systems, steel covered fire extinguishers, radar and television sets, cooking ranges and refrigerators the distance should be not less than 1 m.

The harbour tests given in the section on finding deviation should be carried out prior to the compass being mounted and the friction and gimbal test should preferably be done onshore. The former should be checked with the compass on each of the four main headings. The efficiency of the compass damping system should be tested at this stage. The card is deflected at least 50° from its settling position with a hand held magnet which is then quickly withdrawn. Some texts lay down that the card should then settle back to the original position in a given number of seconds. With the number of different makes of compass available these days, laying down a fixed period could be misleading. If the card moves back sluggishly and if the friction test proved satisfactory, there may have been a loss of magnetism. Lack of damping will be evident in considerable overswinging and several large oscillations about the settling position followed by smaller movements before the card stops. If in doubt over the result, repeat the test on another compass of the same type and compare the two.

Lastly, ensure that the lubber line is fore and aft. One snag with the bulkhead mounted compass is that it will be slightly out if the bulkhead is curved.

Chapter Six
Coastal Position Finding

But the principal failing occurred in the sailing,
and the Bellman, perplexed and distressed,
said he had *hoped, at least, when the wind blew due East,*
That the ship would not *travel due West.*

                    Lewis Carroll, The Hunting of the Snark

In taking a boat from one place to the next, the rhumb line direction between the two, and probably the distance, is first found from the chart and then the boat's position is checked from time to time to ensure that it is not in danger from reefs, rocks or other hazards.

The various methods of finding approximate and accurate positions when on the coast or in pilotage waters are explained in this chapter. The first, dead reckoning, is so old that the exact meaning of the phrase has been lost. Most historians claim that in the early days of sail when a mariner worked out his position he was deducing or reckoning the vessel's progress and that this 'deduced reckoning', often written in the shortened form 'ded reckoning', was inevitably corrupted to the phrase we know today. Others believe that it originated from the use of the Dutchman's log, where a piece of wood was thrown overboard and the vessel's speed was determined relative to the floating wood which was assumed to be stopped, or *dead*, in the water.

Dead reckoning
Dead reckoning is a forecasting ahead on the chart of the boat's probable position based on the direction of travel (course) and speed in knots. The navigator may dead reckon ahead for a minute, an hour or even longer. The accuracy of the forecast position will depend on how well the course is kept, the accuracy of the boat speed used and other factors largely beyond the navigator's control, such as wind and tidal stream, which may set the boat off its intended track.

The dead reckoning track is laid off on the chart by first setting the parallel rulers to the intended course on the compass rose. One edge of the ruler is then moved to a known position of the boat and the course line is drawn in.

In Fig. 56, a vessel leaves a lighthouse at 1000 on a due east course, speed 4 knots. A distance of 4 miles is measured with a pair of dividers from the latitude scale, and the point 4 miles along the course line is marked. This would be the dead reckoning (or DR) position of the boat after one hour, i.e., at 1100. The boat will move 2 miles in half an hour and this distance has been marked along the course line to give the 1130 DR position. The following courses and distances are also shown on the diagram (see Fig. 56):

Time	Course	Speed	Distance
1130 to 1200	180°T	4 kn	2M
1200 to 1240	140°T	6 kn	4M
1240 to 1310	270°T	6 kn	3M

The diagram to this point shows the DR track from the vessel departing the lighthouse at 1000 to the forecast position at 1310. The boat may not be exactly at the position shown, but it is the best information available at that time.

If the navigator decides to return to the starting point at 1310, the course to steer can be found by joining the DR position and the lighthouse as shown. The course would be 312°T, distance 7.5 miles. It would take 1 hour and 15 minutes to cover the distance at 6 knots and arrival time would be 1425. This is called an estimated time of arrival or ETA. It is estimated because it is based on a dead reckoning track, and a further dead reckoning or forecasting ahead. The more proficient the navigator becomes at plotting courses and reckoning ahead, the more accurate will his ETAs become.

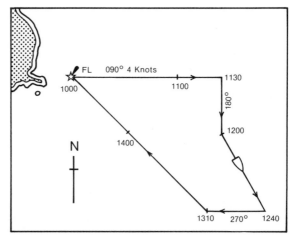

Fig. 56 *A dead reckoning track*

71

						knots								
min	3	3.5	4	4.5	5	5.5	6	7	8	9	10	11	12
2	0.1	0.1	0.2	0.2	0.2	0.2	0.2	0.2	0.3	0.3	0.3	0.4	0.4
4	0.2	0.3	0.3	0.3	0.3	0.4	0.4	0.5	0.5	0.6	0.7	0.7	0.8
6	0.3	0.4	0.4	0.5	0.5	0.6	0.6	0.7	0.8	0.9	1.0	1.1	1.2
8	0.4	0.4	0.5	0.6	0.6	0.7	0.8	0.9	1.0	1.2	1.3	1.5	1.6
10	0.5	0.6	0.7	0.8	0.8	0.9	1.0	1.2	1.3	1.5	1.7	1.8	2.0
12	0.6	0.7	0.8	0.9	1.0	1.1	1.2	1.4	1.6	1.8	2.0	2.2	2.4
14	0.7	0.8	1.0	1.1	1.2	1.3	1.4	1.6	1.9	2.1	2.3	2.6	2.8
16	0.8	1.0	1.1	1.2	1.3	1.5	1.6	1.9	2.1	2.4	2.7	2.9	3.2
18	0.9	1.1	1.2	1.4	1.5	1.7	1.8	2.1	2.4	2.7	3.0	3.3	3.6
20	1.0	1.2	1.4	1.5	1.7	1.8	2.0	2.3	2.7	3.0	3.3	3.7	4.0
22	1.1	1.3	1.5	1.7	1.8	2.0	2.2	2.6	2.9	3.3	3.7	4.0	4.4
24	1.2	1.4	1.6	1.8	2.0	2.2	2.4	2.8	3.2	3.6	4.0	4.4	4.8
26	1.3	1.5	1.8	2.0	2.2	2.4	2.6	3.0	3.5	3.9	4.3	4.8	5.2
28	1.4	1.7	1.9	2.1	2.3	2.6	2.8	3.3	3.7	4.2	4.7	5.1	5.6
30	1.5	1.8	2.0	2.3	2.5	2.8	3.0	3.5	4.0	4.5	5.0	5.5	6.0
32	1.6	1.9	2.2	2.4	2.7	2.9	3.2	3.7	4.3	4.8	5.3	5.9	6.4
34	1.7	2.0	2.4	2.6	2.9	3.1	3.4	4.0	4.5	5.1	5.7	6.2	6.8
36	1.8	2.1	2.4	2.7	3.0	3.3	3.6	4.2	4.8	5.4	6.0	6.6	7.2
38	1.9	2.2	2.6	2.9	3.2	3.5	3.8	4.4	5.0	5.7	6.3	7.0	7.6
40	2.0	2.4	2.7	3.0	3.3	3.7	4.0	4.7	5.3	6.0	6.7	7.3	8.0
42	2.1	2.5	2.8	3.2	3.5	3.9	4.2	4.9	5.6	6.3	7.0	7.7	8.4
44	2.2	2.6	3.0	3.3	3.7	4.0	4.4	5.1	5.9	6.6	7.3	8.0	8.8
46	2.3	2.7	3.1	3.5	3.8	4.2	4.6	5.4	6.1	6.9	7.7	8.4	9.2
48	2.4	2.8	3.2	3.6	4.0	4.4	4.8	5.6	6.4	7.2	8.0	8.8	9.6
50	2.5	2.9	3.4	3.8	4.2	4.6	5.0	5.8	6.7	7.5	8.3	9.1	10.0
52	2.6	3.1	3.5	3.9	4.3	4.8	5.2	6.1	6.9	7.8	8.7	9.5	10.4
54	2.7	3.2	3.6	4.1	4.5	5.0	5.4	6.3	7.1	8.1	9.0	9.9	10.8
56	2.8	3.3	3.8	4.2	4.7	5.1	5.6	6.5	7.5	8.4	9.3	10.2	11.2
58	2.9	3.4	3.9	4.4	4.8	5.3	5.8	6.8	7.7	8.7	9.7	10.6	11.6
60	3.0	3.5	4.0	4.5	5.0	5.5	6.0	7.0	8.0	9.0	10.0	11.0	12.0

Fig. 57 *Time, speed, distance table*

Fig. 57 shows a time, speed and distance table. This is used for finding the distance a boat will travel in a given time up to one hour (60 minutes) at any speed from 3 to 12 knots. For example, the navigator may want to know how far a craft will travel in 20 minutes at 5 knots. Using the table, under 5 knots in the top line and opposite 20 in the minutes column, the distance is 1.7 miles. The table can also be used to find speed, if one knows how far a boat has moved in a given time. First find the correct time in the minutes column. Then go along the line horizontally opposite to find the distance in the main part of the table, and move vertically up that column to read off speed. For instance, to find speed if a boat travels 2.7 miles in 40 minutes, opposite 40 in the left hand column, 2.7 is under 4 in the top line, so the boat's speed is 4 knots.

Okay, so yachts don't travel on exact courses at exact speeds. Both may vary with wind shifts and much of the time may be spent in tacking. For the moment, it is enough to understand what dead reckoning is and how DR tracks and positions are plotted.

There is no hard and fast rule as to how often times should be entered on the track. Some people might argue that as the navigator cannot guarantee that course and speed will be maintained, it would surely be easier to fill in the track every so often, based on the actual courses and speeds made good over a period. They miss the point. Dead reckoning not only shows the boat's probable position but also shows if the intended

72

track is a safe one. A forecast track on the chart also means that the boat's position can be seen at a glance and this is most important in an emergency. When the boat is breaking up around you, this is no time to be fooling around with a pair of dividers working out a DR position to send out in your distress message.

Tidal flow
While the dead reckoning track gives a good guide to position, it does not allow for outside influences acting on the vessel. A better forecast position can be found by taking into account tidal flow, ocean current or any other factor that may set the boat off the intended track. Information can be taken from the flood or ebb arrows or the tidal diamonds on the chart, as discussed in Chapter Two. However, before going on with the mechanics of using this information to estimate position, I would like to clear up a point that can cause uncertainty.

If a craft is moving through the water, tidal stream or current does not register on the log. If moored to a jetty or at anchor and stemming the tidal flow, the rush of water under the hull will register. The moment the lines are let go or the anchor raised from the sea bed, the boat is free to drift with the water and the log speed will drop to zero. Imagine, say, a hundred ships spaced over 25 miles of ocean, all stopped but in a 6 knot current. The whole flotilla would be moving in the same direction at 6 knots, as would everything else in or on the sea. If all the ships got under way on different courses at different speeds, the fleet would still be moving *en masse* in the one direction at 6 knots in the current. However, the reading on each vessel's log would be its speed through the water.

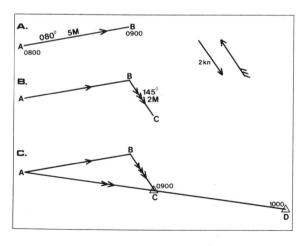

Fig. 58 *Plotting an estimated position. CMG is 097°T and SMG 6.1 kn*

73

Estimated position

A dead reckoning position which is further refined to make allowance for tidal stream or other outside influence on a vessel's progress is said to be an estimated position. For example, a boat heading in an easterly direction with a tidal stream setting to the south-east would be set off the intended track to the south-east. In this case the most probable position after one hour can be found as illustrated in Fig. 58. The course is 080°T, speed 5 knots. The tidal stream is setting 145°T at 2 knots (ebb stream arrow).

Mark the DR track for one hour (line AB in the diagram). From B lay off the direction and distance of the tidal stream for one hour (line BC). C is the estimated position after one hour. The boat will have moved along the line AC, which is called the course made good (CMG). The length of AC is the speed made good (SMG) in one hour. If there is no change in the direction and speed of the boat and the tidal stream, the estimated position (EP) after two hours would be the extension of the line for the distance CD equal to AC − the SMG. By using the speed made good, the navigator can work out the EP at any time along the course made good.

Leeway

If a vessel lies stopped in the water, it will be blown downwind. This effect is still present when moving through the water, but is masked by

Fig. 59 *Leeway*

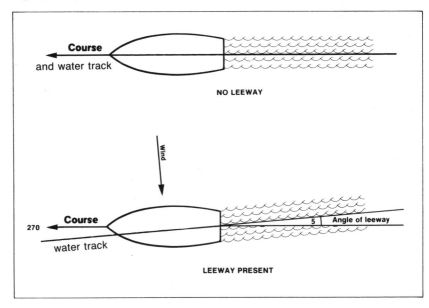

the boat's own speed. This sideways movement through the water caused by a wind on the beam is called *leeway*. Leeway can be estimated by checking the angle between the fore and aft line of the boat and the wake going out astern of the craft. If there is no leeway, the wake will be in a straight line directly astern. The amount of leeway can vary with different sail combinations in the same wind strength, or changes in wind speed with the one set of sails. One method of checking leeway is to choose a position that will probably be part way down the ladder into the cabin, so that when looking aft, the pushpit is level with the horizon. Mark the pushpit or stern rail with tape so that a sighting across the marks shows angles of 5°, 10° and 15° on the port and starboard quarters. The marks and wake will be at the same level when using the same vantage point at sea. The leeway angle can be read off directly if the wake is in line with one of the marks, or estimated if it falls in between.

Leeway can be taken into account when plotting an estimated position by applying the angle to the *true* course being steered. This course with leeway applied is called the *water track*. The boat will be set downwind, as in Fig. 61, but leeway has no effect on speed through the water.

Tidal stream and leeway

When a boat is in a tidal stream and also making leeway, the estimated position is found in two steps, strictly in the following order:

1. Apply the leeway downwind of the true course being steered to find the water track, and plot the resulting course on the chart. Mark off one hour of boat speed along the line.

2. Lay off the tidal stream from the point just plotted to find the EP.

For example, a boat on course 080°T, speed 5 knots is making 8° in a northerly wind. A tidal stream is setting 145°T at 2 knots.

Course steered	080°T
Leeway angle	+8°
Course through the water	088°T (water track)

In Fig. 62, AB is the track for one hour, and BC the tidal stream. C is the estimated position after one hour. The line AC gives the course and speed made good.

Counteracting tidal stream

Although the probable position and future track can be found using the constructions given earlier for plotting estimated positions, there may be times when it is essential to make good a given course regardless of tidal stream effect. Look at Fig. 60. The boat starts at point S, log speed 5 knots, and has to make good a course of 040°T to pass safely between the charted rocks. The tidal stream is setting 310°T at 2 knots.

The course to steer to counteract tidal stream is found as follows. Draw in the intended track. From S, lay off the tidal stream for one hour.

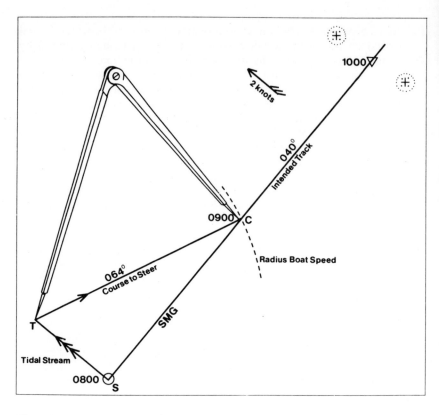

Fig. 60 *Finding course to steer to counteract tidal stream*

Set one hour of boat speed on a pair of dividers or compasses. With centre T, cut into the intended track (point C in the diagram). TC is the course to steer. After one hour, the boat should have reached point C on the intended track, having moved along the line SC on the chart which is the course made good. The distance from S to C is the speed made good in one hour. If the boat course, speed and tidal stream remain unchanged, the craft will continue on the same CMG at the SMG. As these are a combination of both boat and tide movement, any forecasting ahead gives an estimated position. In this example the SMG is 4.6 knots. At this speed the boat should pass between the rocks at 1000.

The slower the boat, the greater the angle of throw-off needed to allow for the same tidal stream. In the above example, the difference between the intended track and the course to steer is 24°. Fig 63 shows that under the same conditions but with a speed of only 4 knots, the throw-off angle would be 30°

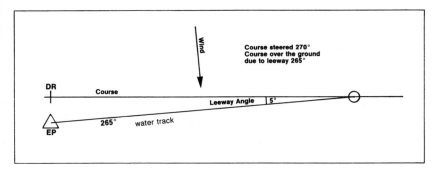

Fig. 61 *Estimated position using leeway angle*

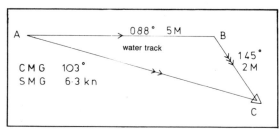

Fig. 62 *Estimated position using leeway angle and tidal stream*

Allowance for leeway

Once the angle has been estimated, leeway can be counteracted by altering by the same amount towards the wind. In Fig. 61 the intended track of 270°T could be made good by altering course to starboard to 275°T.

The course to steer to counteract effects of both tidal stream and leeway is found by first plotting the course to allow for tidal stream, as in Fig. 60, and turning onto it. Once the navigator has estimated the leeway on his heading, the course is adjusted towards the wind. Be very careful here. This true course must then be converted to a compass course to steer. It would be wrong, for example, to turn onto a course to counteract tidal stream, find that the boat was making 10° leeway, and then simply alter the compass course by 10° into the wind. For example, if in Fig. 60 the boat were making 3° leeway in a southerly wind while on course 064°T, the heading would be changed to 064° + 3° or 067°T. In Fig. 63, if a northerly wind was causing 5° leeway, the boat would be brought left to 070° − 5° or 065°T.

In practice the tidal stream changes both direction and speed as time passes and if the boat is in the vicinity of underwater dangers the tidal triangle may have to be redrawn every hour. This requirement can be avoided on a short coastal passage through open water if there is a tide change at about the midway stage and a consequent reversal in the direction of the tidal stream. The direct course could be steered throughout because the boat would be set off track by the last of one stream and back on again by the next. The total time taken on passage

77

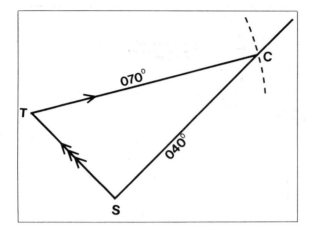

Fig. 63 *The course taken to counteract the tidal stream (070°T) in the slower boat. It then happens that the slower boat has to 'throw off' 30°, compared with the 24° of the faster boat in Fig. 60.*

would be less than it would have been if the navigator had counteracted the stream throughout.

If the tidal stream will be setting in the same general direction during the whole of a passage, and again assuming that there are no dangers close to the track, the navigator can counteract the effects by finding just one average course to steer.

In Fig. 64, a boat is going from S to T. The direct track is 120°T, distance 15 miles. The boat speed is 5 knots so the passage will take about 3 hours. The navigator estimates that during this time the tidal stream will set 045°T at 2.4 knots, 030°T at 1.8 knots and 010°T at 1.3 knots in the first, second and third hours. These directions and distances are laid off from the starting point as shown, and the line SC represents the total drift due to the effects of tidal stream during the first three hours. The boat will travel 15 miles in this time. Set the distance on the dividers and, using point C as the centre, cut into the direct track. The line CD is the course to steer − 140°T − and the boat should have reached D after three hours, a distance made good of 14.5 miles. If the dividers will not open out to the distance steamed, the course can still be found by halving all the distances, i.e., in the above example by using 1.2, 0.9 and 0.65 miles for the tidal streams and 7.5 miles for the distance, it will be found that the course to steer remains 140°T.

Position finding
The dead reckoning and estimated positions are good guides to progress and they may be correct, but the vessel's true position must be found from time to time.

The position line
The basis for finding a boat's position is the position line: *A position line is a line on the chart on which the boat lies or has lain.* It may be

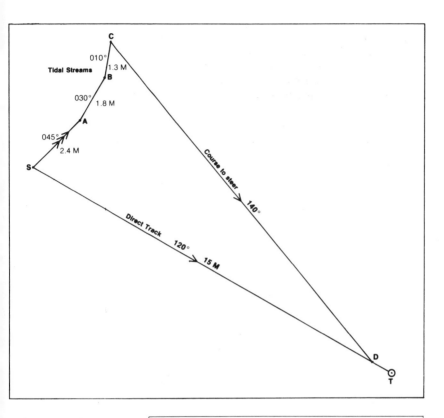

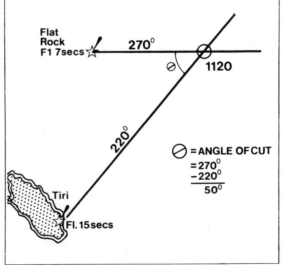

Fig. 64 *Finding course to steer to allow for changing tidal stream*

Fig. 65 *Cross bearing fix showing angle of cut*

straight, curved, or irregular in shape. If two position lines are obtained at the same time, as the vessel lies somewhere on each line the true position must be the point at which the two lines cut.

Finding two or more position lines is called *fixing the boat's position*. The most common method of fixing is by taking simultaneous compass bearings of two prominent charted objects such as lighthouses.

Look at Fig. 65. By using a hand bearing compass as explained on page 83, and adjusting for magnetic variation, the navigator has found

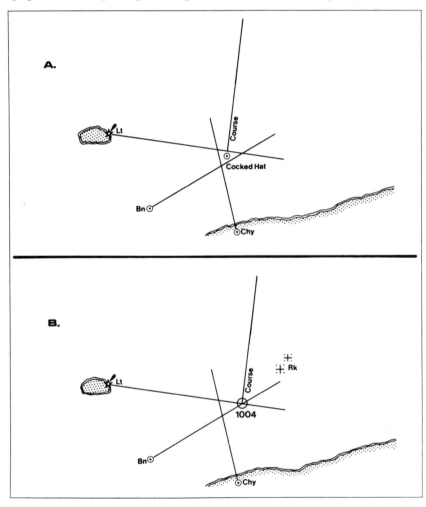

Fig. 66 a *Cocked hat fix* b *Using the most dangerous corner of a cocked hat fix*

that the bearings of Flat Rock and Tiri Light are 270°T and 220°T respectively. The fix is identified by a circle where the bearing lines cross and the time is noted.

Taking the bearings is not always easy and in a pitching or rolling boat, the results may be slightly inaccurate. To overcome this problem, it is usual to take three bearings and if there is an error in one or more of the lines, they will not cross at the same point. The resulting small triangle is called a *cocked hat*, as shown in Fig. 66. The true position is taken as being the centre of the cocked hat. If the boat is close to a danger, to err on the safe side the point closest to the danger is taken as being the position, as in Fig. 66b.

The most accurate fix by two cross bearings is made when the position lines are at right angles to one another because any error in each line has the least effect on the accuracy of the plotted position. The smaller of the two pairs of angles between any two position lines is called the *angle of cut* and is illustrated in Fig. 65. The minimum angle of cut acceptable to get a reliable fix is 30°, especially if only two bearings are taken. The object whose bearing is changing most rapidly, which will

Fig. 67 *Plotting symbols. No official plotting symbols have been laid down, but those shown here have been used by many navigators over the years.*

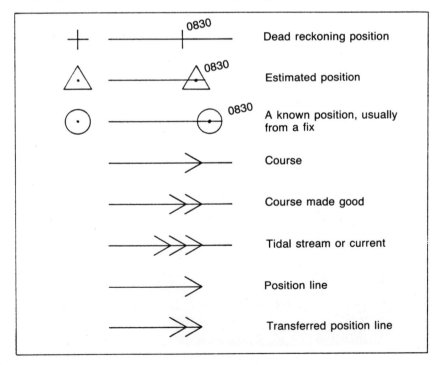

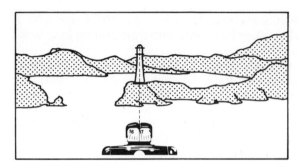

Fig. 68 *Using a hand bearing compass. The bearing of the lighthouse is 168°C.*

be the one closest to the boat and on or near the beam, should be taken last. Use this moment as being the time of the fix. This overcomes the practical problem of not being able to take the bearings at exactly the same time.

Dead reckoning, estimated positions, and two or three bearing fixes together form the basis of keeping a charted plot of the boat's position and track, although there are many and varied ways of fixing. Many of these are discussed shortly, and the majority depend on the use of bearings of charted objects. Before going on with the details of these fixes, I shall examine the practical use, errors, and types of hand bearing compass (see page 11).

THE HAND BEARING COMPASS

Most fixed steering compasses are so placed that it is impossible to get an all-round view of the horizon and coastline because the control panels and/or the boat's superstructure block the way. An essential instrument for use in coastal navigation is the hand bearing compass (HBC) which was illustrated on page 11. As the name implies, it is portable and is mainly

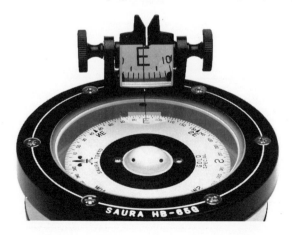

Fig. 69 *Prism sight*

used for taking bearings of shore navigation marks when finding the boat's position. The compass is fitted with a sighting device, usually consisting of a prism that reflects the graduations on the compass card, and a notch or V sight as is found on some rifles. An internal light may be fitted beneath the card, powered by batteries in the compass handle, which illuminates the graduations for use at night.

To use a hand bearing compass, the instrument is held up to eye level and the card is allowed to settle. The prism is adjusted so that the reflection of the figures on the card can be clearly seen when looking horizontally across the bowl. The notch on the top of the prism, the engraved line on top of the bowl and the navigation mark or other object are then all lined up. The reading against the line is the compass bearing of the mark, as shown in Fig. 68.

Choice of instrument

There are many makes of reliable hand bearing compasses: the Sestrel, Danforth White, Finland's Suunto, and the Japanese Saura are trade names that readily come to mind. In general, the larger the model, the more accurate it will be, and the bolder graduations are easier to read, especially in poor light, than those on the smaller compasses. As the HBC is essentially a bearing taker, whatever sort is chosen should be graduated in the circular notation 0°–360°.

One popular model, the mini-compass, is illuminated by a Betalight or self-glowing inbuilt luminous substance. As no batteries are needed, it is very compact, and light enough to be worn around the neck or carried in a pocket when moving around the boat. It has no V sight or hairlines, but is designed so that the graduations are clear with the human eye focused at infinity. The compass can therefore be held close to the eye

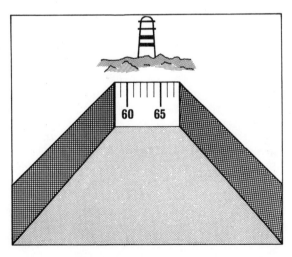

Fig. 70 *View through a mini-compass. The lighthouse bears 063 °C.*

while both the readings and the navigation mark remain in sharp focus. Even without a datum line, the central reading, and thus the bearing of the object, is quite obvious.

Deviation

If the hand bearing compass were used from the same position as the steering compass it would be subject to the same deviating forces, but being smaller it might have greater errors induced in it than those of the larger compass. If held within a metre of the fixed compass, it could have other errors induced by the magnets in the steering compass itself. However, if the HBC is used from any position on deck away from the boat's magnetic influences and those from engines, steel wire rigging or other metallic fittings, it should be free of deviation.

Don't forget about unseen electrical fittings. I once steadied myself against the cabin housing while using the instrument, and couldn't figure out why there was an obvious 10° to 15° error in the compass until I looked on the other side of the panel. A portable VHF set that was going full blast had been hung on the other side, and wood doesn't screen out magnetic influences.

Use in adverse conditions

Taking a bearing with an HBC is relatively easy in calm seas, but at other times the beginner may strike some problems that can be annoying, to say the least. A few tips on how to overcome some of these may be helpful to the reader.

In heavy seas the card on any type of hand bearing compass may not steady up completely but may swing a few degrees from one side to the other. For example, the reading may vary from 050°C to, say, 056°C. Taking the median result — 053°C — should give the bearing accurate to a degree. Again at night in bad weather, some beginners may find it difficult to take the bearing of a light that flashes only once every 20 or 30 seconds. By the time the compass is lined up and steadying, the light has gone out and the temptation is to put the compass down in disgust and wait for the next flash. Then when it does flash — and 30 seconds can seem an eternity at such times — the helmsman has sheered off course, the light comes up where it was least expected, and the dreary process starts again. The solution is to get the rough bearing the first time, if only to the nearest ten degrees, then not to lower the compass but to keep looking along that bearing no matter what the movement of the boat is. When the light flashes again the compass is already steady, and a very slight movement, a few degrees one way or the other, allows the navigator to take the correct reading.

With a little experience it is also possible to get accurate results by taking the bearing of where the light *was* when it went out. That isn't as silly as it sounds, but it does need some practice. Although there are probably very few occasions on which the navigator cannot get a clear field of view by moving around the boat when using a portable compass, on those boats fitted with fixed compasses that have a sighting device, a navigation mark or other object can be blocked by superstructure or sails at a vital moment. Do not despair. Jig around a bit, looking first at the mark to get its position in your mind's eye, and then back again a few times, and take a bearing of that bit of the sail or other structure in line with it.

This procedure is not recommended in heavy weather, when the in-line point may suddenly become an out-of-line point as the boat lurches, but at other times it can be an effective solution. While it is permissible for the navigator to yell politely at the rest of the crew, if the skipper's skull is in the way, don't invite him to pull his woolly head in. Take a bearing of his left or right earhole. In the cases discussed above, any slight error in bearing will show up as a small cocked hat in the fix.

One last point. If a small island is some distance away, it is more accurate to take a bearing of the centre of the island than either of the two edges.

The running fix
Although a fix is usually described as being the point of cut of two or more position lines taken almost simultaneously, there are occasions when only one navigation mark is visible. This happens by day on a featureless coastline or by night when lighthouses are spaced well apart and only one light is visible at any given time.

An approximate position can be found with the one object by using a running or transferred position line fix. To do this, take a bearing and plot it on the chart, then wait until the bearing has changed by a minimum of 30°. Take and plot a second bearing. In both cases, note the time

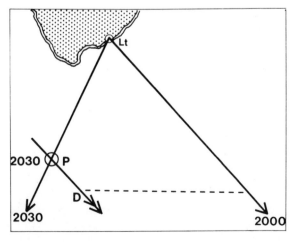

Fig. 71 *Running fix. Course 270°T, speed 4 knots. Distance run between 2000 and 2030 is 2 miles.*

and the log reading. Comparing these readings gives the distance travelled between the two times, and the boat's course is known. The first position line is transferred in the same direction and for the same distance that the boat has moved between the times of taking the two bearings. The point of intersection between the transferred line and the second line is the fix.

Look at Fig. 71. Bearings of the light were taken at 2000 and 2030 and plotted as shown. Then from any point — I'll repeat that, from *any* point on the first line — lay off the boat's course. Mark the distance travelled along it, point D in the diagram. Align the parallel rulers to the first line and transfer it through the point D. The point of intersection, P, is the fix at 2030. However, unknown factors such as bad steering, log error and especially tidal stream effect have not been allowed for, and if in strong tidal waters the running fix should be used only as a *guide* to position. Even so, it is very much better than an inaccurate DR.

A position line should not be transferred more than once because any slight error in the line would be carried forward each time it was moved. If a third bearing of the light were taken at 2115, the 2030 position line would be transferred to give the running fix at 2115, as shown in Fig. 72.

I believe that a major problem for the beginner when learning coastal navigation is that he or she ends up with too many lines drawn all over the chart. When this happens the picture becomes confused, and attempting to understand the procedure being explained becomes very difficult. A cardinal rule in chartwork is: erase all unnecessary lines as you go along.

Doubling the angle on the bow
The emphasis here is not on the use of true bearings but on the change of angle of a shore mark relative to the bow *when the boat is on a steady*

Fig. 72 *Transferring the most recent bearing line*

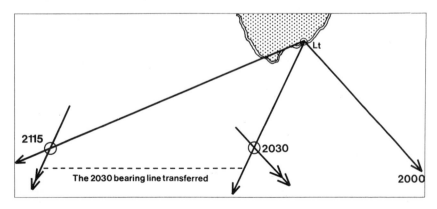

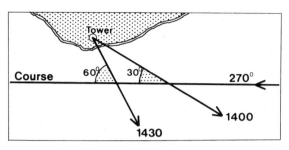

Fig. 73 *Doubling the angle on the bow*

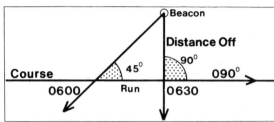

Fig. 74 *Four-point bearing*

course. Fig. 73 shows that at 1400 a tower is 30° on the bow and by 1430 this angle has doubled to 60°. The triangle in the diagram is made up of the two bearings and the boat's track between 1400 and 1430. According to the principles of plane geometry, in this triangle two of the sides are equal in length, i.e., the 1430 bearing and the track. In other words, the boat's distance from the tower at 1430 is equal to the distance run between the times of the two bearings. By doubling any initial angle on the bow (of 30° or more) the distance travelled by log is the distance of the boat from the mark at the time of the second bearing. If the true bearing of the mark is laid off on the chart and this distance marked along it, a fix is obtained.

Four-point bearing

This traditional fix is a special case of doubling the angle on the bow. Older magnetic compasses were divided into 32 points which meant that there were 11¼° in each point. If a fixing mark is 45° (four points) on the bow and the course is maintained until the object is 90° on the bow, i.e., abeam, again the distance off the mark can be found without calculation because it is equal to the distance run between the times of the two bearings, which can be read directly off the log. As the mark is on the beam, the bearing is changing most rapidly and the time of the fix can be judged more accurately than it can be when doubling any old angle on the bow.

Another factor is that the chosen mark does not have to be shown on the chart. The boat's distance off the shoreline passing by on the beam is given by using any convenient mark such as a prominent rock, a

87

conspicuous scar on the cliff face or a tree on the cliff edge, as long as both bearings are taken of the same object.

Caution: Although the fixes for doubling the angle on the bow are convenient, they should never be used if there is any appreciable cross-tide or if the boat is making much leeway. Although it might seem that the four-point fix would be accurate if an unknown tidal stream were running either directly with or directly against the boat, this is not the case. The former would give a position too close to the object observed, while the latter would give a position too far away from the shore mark that was used.

Transferring any position line

A running fix is not limited to using two bearings of the same object. The bearing of one navigation mark can be transferred to the time of finding another bearing from a different mark, and the point at which

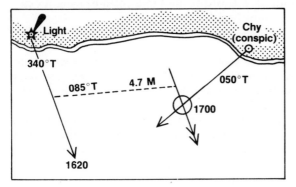

Fig. 75 *Transferring the bearing of one mark to give a fix with the bearing of another*

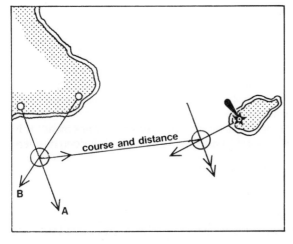

Fig. 76 *Transferring one line of a cross-bearing fix*

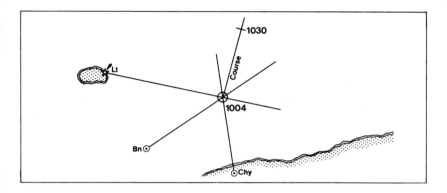

Fig. 77 *Good three-bearing fix and DR track*

the two cut is the fix. Indeed, one of the lines in a cross-bearing fix can be transferred to give a running fix.

The first case is illustrated in Fig. 75. Here a lighthouse was bearing 340°T at 1620. Forty minutes later it was no longer visible but a conspicuous chimney had been sighted bearing 050°T. The boat, which was on course 085°T at speed 7 knots, travelled 4.7 miles between 1620 and 1700. The bearing of the light has been transferred to give the position shown at 1700.

Fig. 76 gives an example of the second case. Here the navigator had obtained a cross-bearing fix, but these marks were lost to view before he sighted the lighthouse. The bearing line marked A has been transferred to give the fix because it gives a good angle of cut. B would make a poor angle of cut with the bearing from the light, leading to an inaccurate position.

Note: At this stage, the reader may think that a fix is where the boat is. It isn't. It's where the boat *was*. Once the bearings are taken, they have to be plotted on the chart. An expert can plot three bearings in about 45 seconds, but until the beginner is proficient in using the parallel rulers it may take up to two or three minutes before the position lines are drawn in. Thus, with either expert or beginner, the resulting point of intersection or fix is history. If it is a cocked hat fix, additional time may be needed to interpret it.

Granted, in open water with the nearest danger some miles away, this fact is not too significant. But in shoal waters and close to hidden dangers the navigator's first concern should not be where he was, or even is, but where he is going to be in the immediate future. Plotting the fix does not finish until a dead reckoning track based on the fix is laid off on the chart, and the navigator is satisfied that the boat is quite safe on its present course, as shown in Fig. 77.

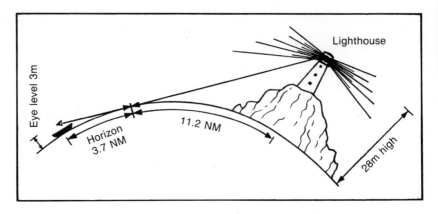

Fig. 78 *Geographical range of a light*

Extreme range fix

One method of finding an approximate position is based on the distance at which a light first appears above the horizon when approaching land, called raising a light, or disappears (dips) below the horizon when leaving the coast. In theory the maximum distance a powerful light can be seen across the curve of the earth's surface on a clear night depends on the height of both the light and the eye of the observer above sea level. This is called the *geographical range* and was given as the visibility of lights on the older fathom charts, assuming the observer's height of eye to be 4.6 m (15 ft). This extreme range is found by adding the distance from the observer to the horizon and the distance from the horizon to the light, as shown in Fig. 73. The two distances can be found by using a table called 'Distance of the sea horizon' contained in any set of nautical tables, or alternatively the total distance can be taken directly from a geographical range table. The tables are entered with the elevation of the light and the observer's height of eye.

For example, an observer whose height of eye is 3 m raises a light with a charted height of 28 m. Using the sea horizon table, the range is found to be 14.9 miles, i.e.:

Distance of boat from horizon (height of eye 3 m)	3.7 miles
Distance from light to horizon (elevation 28 m)	11.2 miles
Distance from boat to light	14.9 miles

Using the geographical range table, under 3 m in the top line and opposite 28 m in the elevation column, the distance is 14.3 miles. The fact that the answer here differs by 0.6 of a mile is of no consequence, as the reader will see shortly.

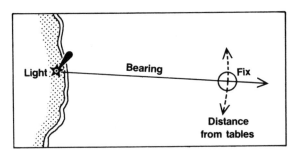

Fig. 79 *Extreme range fix*

A position can be plotted by laying off on the chart the bearing of the light taken on first sighting or just prior to losing it. Mark off the distance from the light along the line of bearing to give the fix.

However, there are certain limitations in the extreme range fix. The method can only be used in clear weather when the loom of the light is visible before the light is raised or after the light dips below the horizon. Under conditions of abnormal refraction, indicated by mirage effects, the actual dipping ranges may increase. Consequently, ranges obtained in this manner should be treated as approximations. The method cannot be used if the charted visibility of the light is less than the geographical range from the tables, because the particular light is not bright enough to be seen along the maximum line of sight distance.

Another factor is that the height of lights is given above the level of mean high water springs. At times other than high water, the amount the tide is below this level should be added to the elevation of the light before entering either of the tables. Naturally the error caused by ignoring this correction depends on the heights of the observer and the light, the tidal range and the time either side of high water. It will be at its greatest at low water and could be over a mile.

Furthermore, in a small boat it is hard to judge the precise time at which a light comes into view or disappears from it, especially with a heavy sea running when the observer's height of eye may change by a

Fig. 80 *Distance of the sea horizon*

Height in metres	Distance in miles	Height in metres	Distance in miles
1	2.1	12	7.3
2	3.0	14	7.9
3	3.7	16	8.5
4	4.2	18	9.0
5	4.7	20	9.5
6	5.2	22	9.9
7	5.6	24	10.4
8	6.0	26	10.8
9	6.4	28	11.2
10	6.7	30	11.6

couple of metres as the vessel rises and falls in the swells.

There seem to be so many restrictions on the use of this method of finding position that the reader may wonder whether it is worth the effort, and what sort of reliance can be placed on the accuracy of the fix. Perhaps a different mental approach should be used by accepting that the position found is approximate and acting accordingly. For example, a navigator who has been unable to fix his position for some time may suspect that his dead reckoning position could be up to 5 miles in error, i.e., the boat could be anywhere inside a circle of uncertainty − centred on the DR as shown in Fig. 82. He sights an expected light on the horizon, bearing 080°T, and according to the tables the range is 16 miles. Assuming this distance to be in error by, say, plus or minus 1 mile he plots the bearing on the chart and marks off ranges of 15 and 17 miles along the line. Agreed, this is not a fix as usually understood, but the navigator has narrowed the limits of his possible position from a circle of uncertainty which happens to have an area of 78.54 square miles down to the single line AB which is 2 miles long. An experienced navigator would not be content with just this step but would try to improve the limits of his probable position by using his depth finder (see page 100).

Elevation in metres m	Height of eye of observer in metres						
	1	2	3	4	5	6
	Range in sea miles					
1	4.1	4.9	5.5	6.1	6.6	7.0
2	4.9	5.7	6.4	6.9	7.4	7.8
3	5.5	6.4	7.0	7.6	8.1	8.5
4	6.1	6.9	7.6	8.1	8.6	9.0
5	6.6	7.4	8.1	8.6	9.1	9.5
6	7.0	7.8	8.5	9.0	9.5	9.9
7	7.4	8.2	8.9	9.4	9.9	10.3
8	7.8	8.6	9.3	9.8	10.3	10.7
9	8.1	9.0	9.6	10.2	10.6	11.1
10	8.5	9.3	9.9	10.5	11.0	11.4
12	9.1	9.9	10.6	11.1	11.6	12.0
14	9.6	10.5	11.1	11.7	12.1	12.6
16	10.2	11.0	11.6	12.2	12.7	13.1
18	10.6	11.5	12.1	12.7	13.2	13.6
20	11.1	12.0	12.6	13.1	13.6	14.1
22	11.6	12.4	13.0	13.6	14.1	14.5
24	12.0	12.8	13.5	14.0	14.5	14.9
26	12.4	13.2	13.9	14.4	14.9	15.3
28	12.8	13.6	14.3	14.8	15.3	15.7
30	13.2	14.0	14.6	15.2	15.7	16.1

Fig. 81 *Geographical range table*

In Fig. 82, the 50-metre depth contour crosses the bearing line almost at right angles. If there was a steeply shelving bottom, with rapid changes in depth, he would find which half of the line AB he was on according to whether the depth was more than or less than 50 metres.

The moral is that no one fixing method, certainly if of doubtful

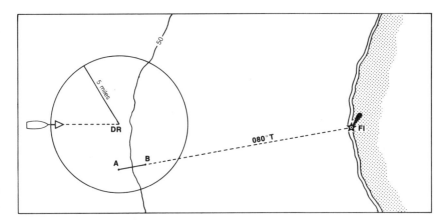

Fig. 82 *Using the extreme range fix to find an approximate position*

accuracy, need be used in isolation. The navigator should at least consider trying to confirm the results obtained by one means by using, as they say, every trick in the book.

Frequency of fixes

The texbooks tell us that when coasting well offshore the position should be checked hourly; if closer in to the coast, perhaps every half hour. When coming into unfamiliar bays and estuaries it may be necessary to fix every fifteen minutes. If the boat is in shoal waters with a strong tidal stream it may be prudent to find position more often.

That's what the textbooks say. Clearly the closer the boat is to hidden dangers, the more vital it is to ensure that the boat is in safe water. This aim may be achieved by using a clearing bearing (page 95) without the need to spend half the time at the chart table plotting fixes every few minutes. On the other hand, even if the boat is well off the coast and fog or bad visibility is threatening, a number of fixes over half an hour may mean the difference between losing the land with an up-to-date position on which to base the subsequent DR or EP, and one which is almost an hour old. The guidelines are fine but the frequency of fixes is dependent on the particular situation.

Having said that, and all else being equal, allowing exactly six minutes between two successive fixes gives a quick and easy check on speed. Six minutes is one tenth of an hour, so the distance between the two fixes in tenths of a mile equals the speed in knots. For example, if a boat travels 0.7 miles in 6 minutes, the speed made good is 7 knots.

Some readers may consider that there is little point in putting positions on the chart when cruising in familiar waters. They may be right, but only with practice comes proficiency in taking bearings and plotting a fix. With proficiency comes confidence that the answers are correct. If

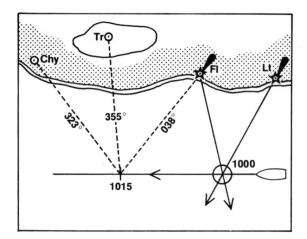

Fig. 83 *Approximate bearings of three marks based on 1015 DR*

the procedure is begun in unfamiliar and perhaps dangerous waters, the navigator may be left with a nagging doubt as to the accuracy of the positions obtained. The place to learn and gain some speed in plotting is in the well-known home cruising ground. Then when one sails further afield one has the calm assurance of knowing what one is doing and, better still, knowing that the fixes are accurate.

Planning ahead

Taking a fix should not be a spur-of-the-moment decision. Identifying navigation marks is not always easy, even in good visibility. Precious time can be wasted in the process and it is quicker in the long run to plan the next fix as soon as the previous one is on the chart. Assume for the moment that the position is being plotted every fifteen minutes. The chart should be inspected to see which marks could be the most useful for the next fix.

The approximate bearings can be found as shown in Fig. 83. Here there is a fix at 1000. By laying off the parallel rulers from the 1015 DR, the navigator can forecast the bearings of three suitable marks accurate to a degree or so. After converting these to magnetic bearings, looking along these bearings with a hand bearing compass shortly before 1015 should aid him in making positive identification of the chosen marks. While it may be convenient to take the bearings at the exact quarter or half hour, a few minutes' delay may mean that a more conspicuous mark is then visible or that the angle of cut has increased from a marginal 30° to a more accurate 35°. The accuracy of a fix is the prime concern, not the convenience to the navigator of the time it is taken.

Set and drift

Dead reckoning was defined earlier as forecasting the boat's probable

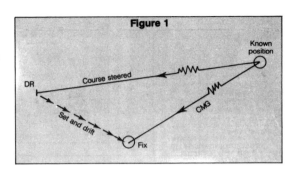

Fig. 84 *Finding unknown tidal stream*

position based on a known start point, using true course and boat speed through the water in knots. Any subsequent fixes should match up with the dead reckoning positions at the times of the fixes. If they do not coincide, and as a fix is where the craft is known to be, then the difference between them must be due to unknown factors which have taken the boat off the dead reckoning track.

This difference can be measured as a direction and distance from the DR position to the known position or fix. The direction which can be measured on the compass rose is called *set*, and the distance in miles is called *drift*. If a boat experiences a drift of 6 miles over a two-hour period then the rate of drift is 3 knots. Finding set and drift gives the navigator a means of establishing the rate and direction of an unknown tidal stream or current (see Fig. 84). For example, if set and drift over a 20 minute period is 090°T, 0.4 miles, then the direction and rate of tidal flow is 090°T, 1.2 knots. This information can be used either to plot accurate estimated positions on the chart or to work out the course to steer to counteract the tide.

Caution: the set and drift procedure must not be used to find current if the boat is making much leeway, because the drift will be made up of both tide and leeway. Nor can the direction and distance from an estimated position to a fix be used to find set and drift. In this situation, the navigator must use boat course and speed to plot a dead reckoning position on the chart and relate this to the fix position.

The clearing bearing

Although fixing is the only way of finding position, knowing where the boat is *not* can be just as useful in some circumstances. For example, if there is one dangerous rock in a bay, to be able to guarantee that the vessel is not too close to it could be as reassuring as knowing the boat's exact position.

Look at Fig. 85. If a boat was approaching Tiri Light from the east, Shearer Rock could be a danger if the boat's position was not known. The dotted line shows that if a vessel was steering 260°T with the light directly ahead, it would hit the rock. On the other hand, if the approach was made along the 280° track, the rock would be passed safely, leaving

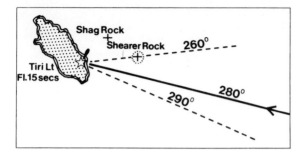

Fig. 85 *Clearing bearing*

it to the north. If the light was on a true bearing of 290°, the vessel would pass even further to the south of the danger.

From this it can be seen that, as along as the bearing of the light is 280°T or *greater*, the vessel must be in safe water. This is true even if the light is not directly ahead, and the 280° line is called a *clearing bearing*, i.e., in using it as above, the vessel will clear the rock safely on the way past (see Fig. 85).

Fig. 86 shows the use of a clearing bearing in the context of avoiding an underwater danger in a bay. The navigator hopes to approach the anchorage along the dotted line but there is no navigation mark directly ahead. However, a clearing line has been drawn in, based on the charted

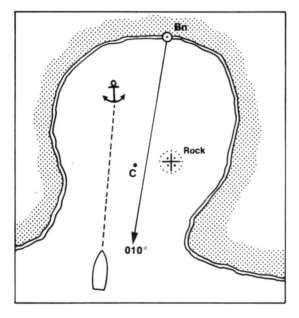

Fig. 86 *Use of a clearing line to enter a bay*

beacon. As long as the beacon bears more than 010°T, the boat must be to the west of the clearing line and in deep water. For example, even if a crosstide drifted the boat to the spot marked C, the beacon would bear 014°T, showing that the boat had not reached the clearing line.

TRANSITS

Any two objects that are in line when seen from a boat are said to be in transit, as explained in Chapter Five. If they are marked on the chart, the craft lies somewhere on the extension of the line joining the two and is a *position line*. Harbour authorities set up pairs of marks that, when kept in transit, lead a ship down the centre of the channel. The rear mark is higher than the front, and each has a distinctive light. A vessel can negotiate the channel by night by keeping these leading lights, as they are called, in transit. The harbour chart shows a line joining the marks with a caption such as: 'Lights in line 142°'. These leading marks have been set up for a specific purpose, but the navigator, by selecting any two charted objects and manoeuvring his boat until they are in line, knows that he is on the seaward side of the line joining the two. If the marks are kept in line, the boat must be moving along the line.

Look at Fig. 87. The line joining the tower and water tank passes north of the sunken rock. The navigator can guarantee to clear the unseen danger as he passes by keeping them in transit.

If a boat is set off the line of a transit there is sometimes a mental block when trying to decide which way to turn to bring the marks back into line. The 'three f's' rule is useful here: *Always follow the front*

Fig. 87 *Use of transit to clear a rock*

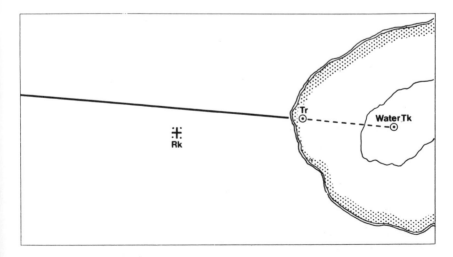

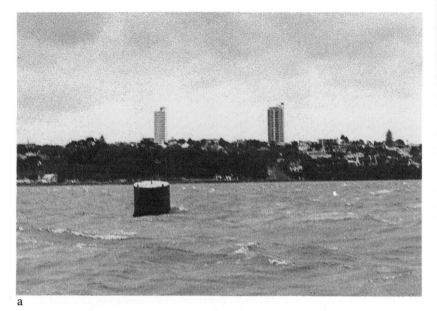

a

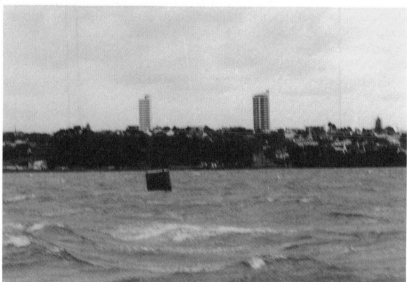

b

Fig. 88 *Now you see it, now you don't. The can-shaped port-hand channel buoy is in line with the left-hand conspicuous building in Fig. 88a. The two marks are no longer in transit in Fig. 88b, although the boat has moved only a few metres. This well-defined moment of transit gives an accurate position line.*

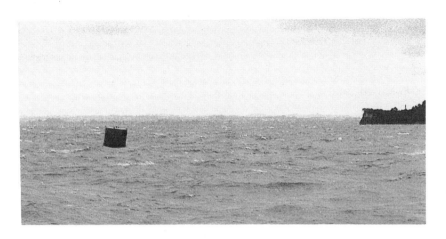

Fig. 89 *Transits: the 'three f's' rule applies*

fellow. In other words, if the front mark is to the left of the rear, go left. For example, in Fig. 89 the buoy is to the left of the steep headland, and the boat should be turned to port to bring these two marks back into line. Try the procedure a couple of times at home, using a pair of lamp posts or any two convenient marks.

A transit can be used in fixing as it gives a position line independent of magnetic variation or any compass error. *However, the distance of the boat from the front mark should not be more than three times the distance between the marks.*

A ship leaving harbour uses the same leading marks as it did when entering but it keeps them in transit astern. Do not fall into the trap of vainly searching the chart for suitable objects ahead while overlooking a perfectly good pair of marks behind the boat.

Measured distance

The extreme accuracy of the moment of transit of two well-defined marks is used in defining a measured distance, usually one nautical mile, for checking speed by log. Two pairs of marks are set up onshore to show each end of the measured mile. Two runs are made over the distance, one in each direction to cancel out the effect of tidal stream. The courses steered are at right angles to the line of the transits. The time taken on each run is noted and the speed by log recorded. The engine should be at the same RPM on each run. The speed on each run is worked out and the two speeds averaged to give boat speed through the water, which is what the log should have been showing. Any difference is converted to a percentage error. This can be used to give speed when using the log for dead reckoning purposes.

For example, say a boat does two runs over the measured mile. The

99

first with the tide takes 8½ minutes, the second against takes 12 minutes. Log speed on both runs is 6.6 knots.

Speed on run 1:		
One mile in 8½ minutes	7	knots
Speed on run 2:		
One mile in 12 minutes	5	knots
Average	12	
	2	
Boat speed through the water	6	knots
Speed by log	6.6	knots

The log is over-reading by 0.6 knot, i.e., 0.6 of a knot in 6 knots or 10 per cent.

In this case, the correct speed is found by multiplying the log speed by $\frac{100}{110}$ i.e.:

$$\frac{6.6 \times 100}{110} = 6 \text{ knots}$$

If the log has been under-reading by 10 per cent, the correct speed is given by multiplying log speed by $\frac{100}{90}$.

For example, if the actual speed is 6 knots the log speed would be 5.4 knots.

$$\text{Boat speed} = \frac{5.4 \times 100}{90}$$
$$= 6 \text{ knots}$$

Using total time and total distance to find the speed is not correct. Assume that the boat speed is in fact 12 knots and that the tide is 6 knots. With the tide against, the boat will take 10 minutes to run the mile because speed made good is 6 knots. When running with the tide, the boat is moving between the marks at 18 knots and would take 3⅓ minutes.

Total distance	2 miles
Total time	13⅓ minutes
Apparent speed	9 knots

Line of soundings

It may be possible to find position by matching a series of soundings with the depths given on the chart. The method can be useful when closing land in fog or thick weather or at night when approaching an unlighted coast. The boat must be kept on a steady heading and the approximate height of tide at the time subtracted from the depth finder readings so that the corrected readings can be compared directly with the depths on the chart.

Fig. 90 *Measured mile*

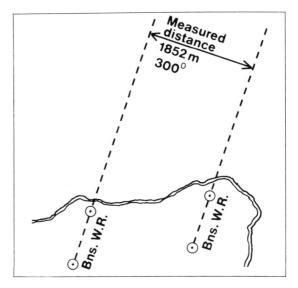

This process is called *reduction to soundings*. The procedure works best where the depths change reasonably rapidly and should not be used where the chart or depth finder shows that there is a flat or gently shelving bottom with little variation in depth.

One method of finding the line of soundings is to note the depth at fixed distances run by log; every quarter, half, or one mile depending on the scale of the chart in use. Another way which is useful if there are sudden and marked variations in depth is to note the time, log reading and depth whenever the sounding changes radically and the difference between successive log readings gives the distance run between soundings.

Alternatively, the distance run between each sounding can be worked out by using the boat speed. Whichever method is used, the distances are measured from the latitude scale of the chart and marked along the edge of a piece of tracing paper. The corrected depths are noted alongside. The edge of the paper is placed on the compass rose and aligned to the course being steered, then moved over the chart surface until the depths noted on the paper match the soundings on the chart. The boat's position at the time that the last sounding was recorded is where it covers the equivalent charted depth. If the navigator has one of those pencils that write on any surface, the depths can be noted on the edge of the parallel rulers instead of on tracing paper. The rulers will stay accurately aligned to the course as they are moved about the chart.

The second method described above is illustrated in Fig. 91. The navigator of a boat which is closing the coast on course 020°T has recorded the details shown in Fig. 91a.

He is hoping to anchor in Sandy Bay and his dead reckoning track is shown. Being prudent, he stops the boat while plotting the information and making the line of soundings match, because this takes several minutes and a glance at the chart shows that with a depth of 14 m he is getting too close to the coast for comfort without knowing his position. In any similar circumstances, the navigator should decide at what stage

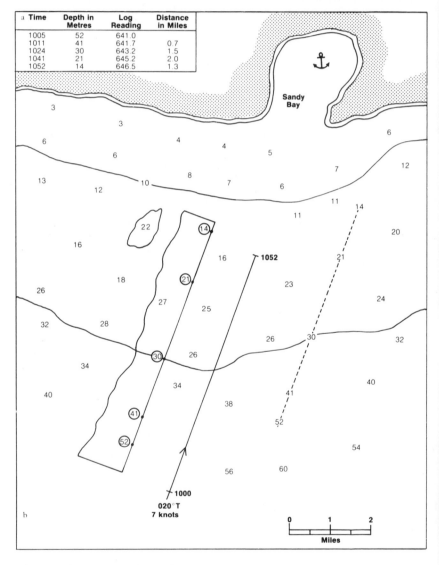

Time	Depth in Metres	Log Reading	Distance in Miles
1005	52	641.0	
1011	41	641.7	0.7
1024	30	643.2	1.5
1041	21	645.2	2.0
1052	14	646.5	1.3

Fig. 91a and b *Line of soundings*

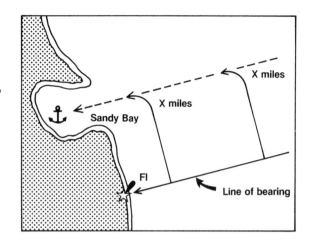

Fig. 92 *Using bearing of the light to choose the moment to turn into the bay*

he must stop and anchor or reverse course back into clear water, rather than blundering on into shallow or dangerous water. This navigator had decided that he would haul off the coast and wait for better visibility if he had not fixed his position by the time of crossing the 10 m depth contour.

Once an accurate comparison is made, the navigator should ensure that the line of soundings cannot be made to fit at any other place on the chart. If it can, the vessel's position remains in doubt. This ambiguity can sometimes be resolved by a bold alteration of course. For example, in the diagram there is a similar set of soundings shown by the dotted line. However, having reached the 14 m depth, if the boat was turned into a due west heading and had been at the circled sounding, the depth would suddenly increase to over 20 m as the boat reached the 22 m hole in the sea bed. On the other hand, if the boat had moved along the dotted line the depth would change to about 11 m and then decrease rapidly as the 10 m line was crossed.

Use of a single position line

A single position line can be put to very good use in certain circumstances. In Fig. 92, the navigator was only able to obtain one bearing on the light prior to losing it and intends to anchor in the bay shown. The line of bearing is along the same bearing that leads into the bay, i.e., parallel to the required track. By running a dead reckoning track at a broad angle — preferably 90° — the navigator can choose the moment to turn and run into the bay. Although the boat's exact position on the line of bearing is not known, running the same distance from any point on the line means that the boat will turn onto the desired track. The same procedure could be used by day if the bearing of the light were taken just as visibility was being reduced by fog or mist.

LOG ...... _Moonsite_ ......

From _Hog Bay_ **to** _Day Cruising_   **Date** _12·20·_   **19_81_**

Time	Log	Miles run	Compass course	Variation	Deviation	True course	Wind	Leeway	CMG	Baro-meter	Temperature Air	Temperature Sea	Speed or RPM
0600	0	2											
0700	5·5	5·5	Various			Various	calm						
0800	11·6	6·1	164°	10°E	3°E	177°	lightair			1020	26°	23°	6 kn
0900	17·5	5·9	116°	10°E	2°E	128°							6 kn
1000	23·5	6·0	211°	10°E	3°E	224°			218°				6 kn
1100	28·7	5·2	293°	10°E	0	303°		5°	308°				
1200	34·1	5·4	"			"	SW4		"	1016	28°	24°	
1300	39·1	5·0	"			"			"				
1400	45·1	6·0	032°	10°E	4°W	038°			034°				
1500	50·1	5·0	"			"			"				
1600	56·7	6·6	018°	10°E	3°W	025°	SW2		020°	1016	26°	24°	6½ kn.
1615	58·1	1·4	Various										

Hour	Latitude	Longitude	Total run		Engine use:
			0530 to 1615		..5¼..Hours
0800	2° 11' N	157° 07'W			
1200	2° 08' N	157° 08' W	...60..miles		Fuel state:

Fig. 93 _Log book and entries_

Deck log

A boat's log is both a diary of events and a record of navigational information. The latter should be in enough detail to permit the boat's track during all or any part of a coastal (or ocean) passage to be fully reconstructed on the chart from the information in the log. The log book itself may consist of a commercially bought hard cover lined volume with pre-printed columns and headings, or even an exercise book ruled up

104

NOTES

0513	Checked HBC. No error	LW 0640 HW 1238
0520	John and Mary Brown on board for day	LW 1810
0530	Up anchor, underway on engine	0601 Sunrise
0630	Course 164° C	0602 No 2 Bn 080° T
0645	Seal rock abeam to port, 3 M	Seal rock 123°
0730	Depth finder on	0746 Seal rock in
0755	Haze obscuring navigation marks.	transit with Spur
0800	Course 116° C - No wind.	point light. Depth 50 m
0902	Course 211° C, light winds. Running on engine.	
1000	Wind increasing from SW. Hoisted main and new genoa	1225 Depth 10 m Cox
1010	Course 293° C 6 kn.	Bank
1250	Heavy rain showers. Visibility 1 to 2 miles	
1255	John Brown slipped - Broken leg? Back to harbour.	
	Radioed ahead for doctor. ETA 1600	
1302	Course 032° C. Hoisted spinnaker	
1400	Depth finder on.	1406 Depth 50 m
1450	Visibility 5 to 10 miles	1500 Bluff light 005° T
1453	Sighted West Bluff light brg. 006° T	Spur Pt. Lt 077° T
	OK well clear of Hope shoal	CMG 1300-1500 034° T
1530	Under power (6½ knots)	
1545	Courses as required to close jetty on brg. 020° T	
1620	Secured alongside Hog Bay jetty. Sloop Blue Crusader alongside.	
	Ambulance waiting, but John's leg not broken - severe strain	
1730	To local yacht club - Christmas party.	
		1803 Sunset

by the navigator to his own requirements. Many people develop their own ideas on the entries needed, and the snag with the pre-printed books is that there are always one or more headings that don't fit in with the user's ideas, or no space for others that do. This snag does not arise if one buys what will be a less expensive book anyway and heads it up oneself, but some people may find the extra work involved a bit of a bore. Even so, my choice is for a decent-sized hard cover book ruled up to the skipper's satisfaction with the headed columns on the left hand page of each opening, and all the right hand page reserved for remarks and narrative entries. This log can be supplemented by two hard back notebooks, preferably pocket size. The navigator can record all bearings, fixes and other data in one of these, and the helmsman enters courses steered, speed and sail changes and any incidents of note while the facts are still fresh in his mind in the other. The navigator, who is usually the one invited to compile the fair log, can transcribe the significant entries from both notebooks on, say, a twice daily basis.

The column headings shown in Fig. 93 are not intended to be exhaustive, but will give the reader a guide to the type of data that should be recorded at regular intervals.

Entries

Time Entries are usually made on the exact hour, but the first entry may be for the time of departure.

Log The distance reading on the log should be reset to zero before leaving the boat's moorings, and then the distance by log entered hourly.

Miles run The difference between each hourly log reading.

Compass course The course the helmsman has been instructed to steer. Where this changes frequently, write 'various' or 'var'. The times of each course change should be transferred from the notebook or notebooks to the remarks page.

Variation The current value of variation, taken from the chart in use.

Deviation Taken from the deviation card for the particular compass course, or deviation of the steering compass, found by use of transits, or other means.

True course The compass course corrected for variation and deviation.

Wind Entered as a direction, and either a force from the Beaufort scale, or the wind speed in knots.

Leeway Best estimate of the angle of leeway, if any.

CMG The course made good after allowing for leeway and/or tidal stream.

Barometer The pressure in millibars. Readings need only be taken every three or four hours but should be entered more frequently if bad weather is in the offing.

The air and sea temperatures can be entered as convenient, but at least four-hourly.

Speed or RPM This column is for use in power boats or yachts proceeding under power.

Notes This page is like the pioneer's stockpot; anything and everything goes in. It should contain changes: of course, speed or RPM if under power, of sail, and in the weather, with times and details. Other entries include departures and arrivals of the craft, all bearings, fixes, sightings of land and other vessels (plus names), and the raising and dipping of lights. Again, times must be included alongside. The log should show the names of crew and visitors on board and all unusual occurrences or emergencies — in short, anything, that will make the document a complete history of the boat and its cruises, and an interesting book to browse through in later years.

Saturday at sea

It is shortly after five o'clock in the morning (navigators don't always go around sounding like Daleks quoting precise times like 05 h 04 m in tinny voices) and a yachtsman is pottering around at the chart table waiting for the day's visitors to come on board. His boat will never win the Americas Cup, but it sails pretty well and the motor isn't as old as all that. Overnight rains have cleared but as yet there is little wind. The 0500 radio weather forecast has promised south-westerly winds, increasing in the late morning, weather fine at first, with possibly some early morning coastal haze. Heavy showers are forecast for the early afternoon, but clearing in the late afternoon or evening. The seas, apparently, will be slight. He checks the tide tables — LW 0640, HW 1238, LW 1810 — before climbing on deck, and as the craft swings to its anchor he notices that No. 1 beacon and the Spur Point light are just coming into line (see Figs 93 and 94). The chart shows that, when in transit, their bearing is 113°M. A sighting with the hand bearing compass shows that it has no deviation, and a comparison between the HBC and steering compass proves that the deviation in the latter tallies with that given on the deviation card. It is always reassuring to know that the compasses have not developed unknown errors.

The traditional rhyme 'outward bound, don't run aground' runs through the skipper's mind, but with the boat carrying the last of the ebb and no shoals or reefs to worry about, there will be no problem leaving this harbour. His friends are on board by 0520, and at 0530 the boat is under way with revs for about 6 knots. A bearing on the conspicuous Sail Rock as No. 2 beacon comes into transit with Spur Point light gives an easy fix on clearing the harbour at 0620. Sail Rock comes abeam at 0645, and as low water is at 0640 the skipper works out that there will be very little tidal stream for a time. A few minutes spent at the chart shows that the boat should cross the 50 m depth contour at 0745.

West Bluff disappears into the haze by 0730 and a few minutes later the depth finder is run up. Allowing for the height of tide, the 50 m line is reached as Sail Rock comes into transit with the Spur Point light, giving the fix shown at 0746. Shortly afterwards, these navigation marks are also lost. The skipper decides to make some ground to the south-east, hoping to use the forecast south-westerly wind later in the day to move back to the north-west with the boat on a broad reach, followed by a spinnaker run back to Hog Bay.

At 0800 course is altered to 128°T, and the tidal arrow shows that the boat will be running directly with any tidal stream. However, on turning to course 218°T a few minutes after nine o'clock, the boat will be set to the south-east by the full force of the flooding tide over the next hour or so. A tidal triangle using 1 knot of tide and a 6 knot boat speed shows that the course to steer to counteract the effect of the tidal stream is 228°T. The skipper plots this construction clear of the boat's track, as shown in Fig. 94. Why not? It's only a triangle, and it doesn't

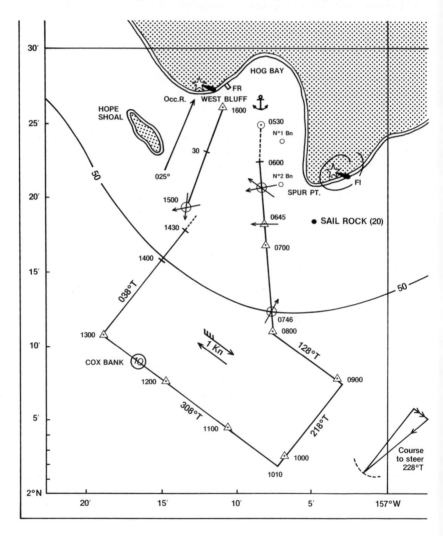

Fig. 94 *A day's cruising, showing the charted track*

matter a shoot where it is drawn. At least the track is kept free from unnecessary and possibly confusing lines, and once the required information, the course to steer and speed made good are found, the triangle can be erased.

The promised wind slowly increases and by 1000 is blowing at about 15 knots from the south. Ten minutes later, and now under sail, the boat is turned to a north-westerly heading. After a few minutes on course 08°T, it is clear from the wake streaming out astern at a slight angle that the craft is making some 5° leeway in a strengthening south-westerly wind and course is adjusted to 303°T to allow for this. From the navigation standpoint, there is not much to do except keep the log up-to-date and plot the hourly EPs on the chart, so the crew settle down to enjoy a few hours in the sun and the wind. The depth finder is switched on at 1215 and ten minutes later the bottom shoals rapidly to 10 m, showing that the boat is over Cox Bank and pretty much on track. Accidents always happen at the least expected times, and the entries in the log (Fig. 93) tell the story.

With the boat on course 038°T and the spinnaker up, the return to harbour is begun at 1300. The 50 m line is crossed on schedule just after 1400 in reduced visibility, but the heavy showers clear towards three o'clock, and the shore navigation marks are sighted. The only danger on this leg is that the boat might be set to the north-west by the start of the ebb, towards Hope Shoal, and the skipper has laid off a clearing bearing on the chart based on the West Bluff light. This is 025°T or less, and as the bearing of the light on first sighting is 006°T, the boat is well to the east of the danger.

A two-bearing fix at 1500 shows that the boat has been set slightly off track by the ebb stream, and by 1530 the wind is easing. The course to make good to close the Hog Bay jetty is 020°T, and course 025°T is being steered to counteract the ebb stream, with the boat now under power. From 1550 onward the jetty itself is used as a leading mark, and course is altered as necessary to keep it bearing 020°T. The estimated time of arrival, based on the fix at 1500, is 1615.

There may be a gap or two in the narrative and the odd coincidence, such as crossing the 50 m line at the exact moment that two navigation marks came into transit, but it gives the reader an idea of the sort of information that is kept on the chart and the types of entries found in the log. Although the complete track is shown in Fig. 94, in practice the past track can be erased from time to time, especially if the boat is criss-crossing the same general stretch of water.

A final hint. When using unfamiliar charts, it can be most frustrating trying to pick out the major navigation marks quickly, especially at night in dim light. Before arriving in the general area, why not circle the marks in pencil, as has been done with the Spur Point light in Fig. 94. It may be ugly, but you can see it in a hurry when you need it.

Chapter Seven
Sextant Fixing

Readers who are only going to be involved in coastal navigation do not need expensive sextants. But the blue water navigator, who must own one, may not realise just how useful it can be in coastal fixing. As the reader in the latter category will know the principles on which it works, and how to use the sextant, no detailed explanation is included here.

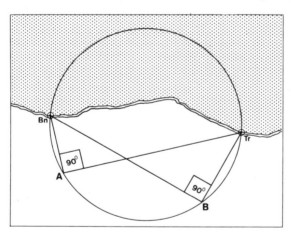

Fig. 95 *A horizontal sextant angle gives a circle of position. The boat lies somewhere on the circumference.*

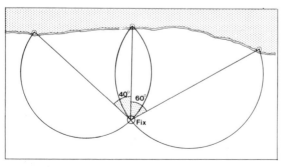

Fig. 96 *HSA fix. The angle between the centre mark and left hand mark as viewed from the boat, called the 'left angle', is 40°. The 'right angle' is 60°. The point of intersection of the two circles is the boat's position.*

Horizontal sextant angles

The angle between any two charted objects in roughly the same horizontal plane can be measured with a sextant, which gives a circle of position or curved position line. Look at Fig. 95. The angle between the tower and the beacon is a right angle or 90° at both points A and B which lie on the circle shown. This circle passes through the two fixing marks and the angle between them is 90° from any point on the circle. For any given angle between the marks, a circle can be drawn passing through the two objects and the observer. If three fixing marks are selected and the angles between the centre mark and each outer mark are measured with a sextant, two

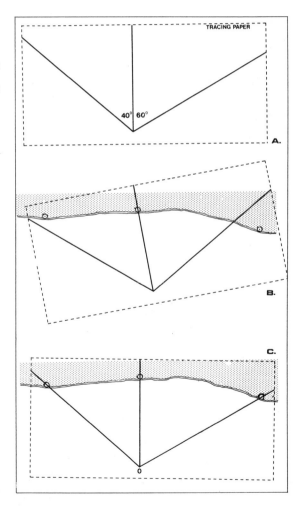

Fig. 97a, b and c
Steps in plotting the fix when the two angles are drawn on tracing paper

111

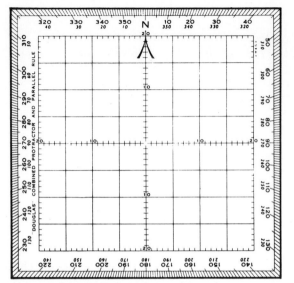

Fig. 98 *Douglas protractor*

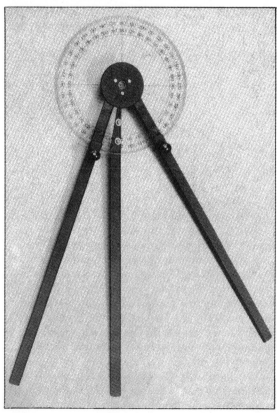

Fig. 99 *Station pointer*

112

position circles are obtained. The point of intersection between the two circles is a fix, as shown in Fig. 96.

Plotting the fix

It is not necessary to plot the two circles on the chart to find the boat's position. The two angles can be drawn on tracing paper, radiating from a common point (O in Fig. 97). The paper is then placed over the chart, with the centre line on the centre object, and adjusted so that each line crosses one of the fixing marks. The boat is at O and the position can be pricked through onto the chart with a point of the dividers.

Horizontal sextant angle (HSA) fixes can also be plotted by using a Douglas protractor, in the same manner as with tracing paper. The engraved north-south line is used as the centre line, and the two angles are drawn in pencil on the matt surface. As the protractor has to be turned over when placed on the chart, the two angles have to be reversed when they are laid off. The larger sized protractor is needed here, because the lines on the smaller model would be too short to reach across the chart to the three fixing marks.

The most accurate method is to use a station pointer. The two outer legs are set at the required angles. The bevelled edge of the fixed centre leg is placed over the centre mark on the chart and the station pointer is adjusted until the bevelled edges of all three legs are over the three fixing marks.

The advantages of the HSA fix are that a very precise position is found because the sextant can be read more accurately than a compass and the fix is independent of magnetic variation or compass error. However, there are disadvantages — three suitable fixing marks must be chosen from

Fig. 100 *Suitable fixing marks*

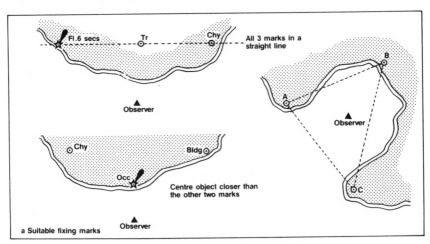

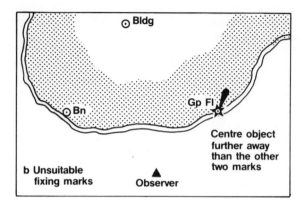

Fig. 101 *Unsuitable fixing marks*

the chart and the fix may take longer to plot than it does using other methods.

Choosing the marks

Any three objects that meet one of the following requirements are suitable for an HSA fix.

1. The marks lie in the one straight line.

2. The centre mark is closer to the boat than the other two.

3. The boat lies inside the triangle formed by the three marks.

Additionally, in any HSA fix the angle between each set of marks should be a minimum of 30°.

If the outer marks are closest to the boat, as in Fig. 101, ambiguity

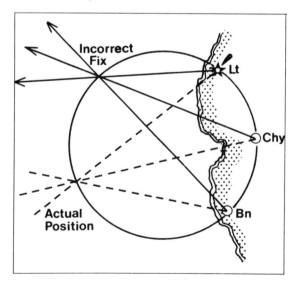

Fig. 102 *If the boat lies on the circle passing through the three objects, the plotted position may be in error because the two angles are the same at any point on the circle.*

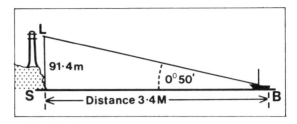

Fig. 103 *Distance by vertical sextant angle*

91·4 m

0° 50'

S ← Distance 3·4 M → B

can arise if the craft is on or near the circle that passes through the three objects. The angles between the marks are the same anywhere on the circle, so the plotted fix may be a point on the circumference that is very different to the true position of the boat.

Vertical sextant angles

The navigator can use a sextant to find his distance from a lighthouse as long as both the light and shoreline directly below it can be seen. In Fig. 103, SB is the distance from below the base of the light to the vessel and is part of the right-angled triangle SLB. The side SL is the height of the light and can be found from the chart or light list. The angle at B, which is the angle between the light and shoreline beneath as seen from the boat, can be measured with a sextant.

Any set of nautical tables will have a section called 'Distance by vertical angle' which gives the distance off using the sextant angle and the height of the object in feet or metres. For example, the tables tell us that for

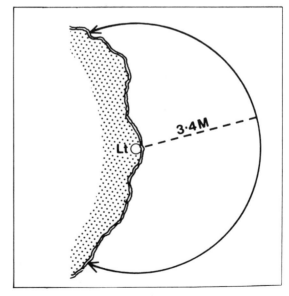

Fig. 104 *Curved position line or range arc*

3·4M

Lt

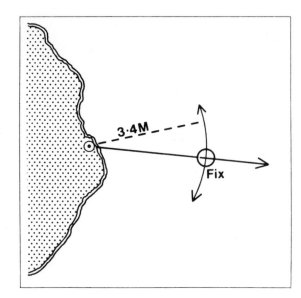

Fig. 105 *Bearing of the light is 276°T. Using VSA range of 3.4 miles gives the boat's position.*

3·4M

Fix

an angle of 0°50′ and a 300 ft (91.4 m) object, the distance is 3.4 miles. With the lighthouse as centre and using a radius of 3.4 miles, a circle or part circle can be drawn on the chart. This known distance from a light gives a curved position line sometimes called a range arc.

There is a bonus in that a bearing of the light can be taken at the same time as the vertical sextant angle. This results in a fix from *only one object* consisting of a bearing and a range arc.

Rule of thumb
If you do not hold a set of tables then you can work out the distance using the following rule of thumb:

$$\text{Distance off in miles} = \frac{\text{Height of light in metres}}{\text{Sextant angle in minutes}} \times 1.86$$

Using a height of 32 m and VSA 0°40′ the distance by tables is 1.5 miles. The answer by rule of thumb is:

$$\frac{32 \times 1.86}{40} = 1.488 = 1.5 \text{ miles}$$

Range arc fix
In Fig. 106, the navigator has used the distances from two lighthouses to give a fix by crossing two range arcs. In practice it would be quicker to use just the one range and a bearing, but in radar-fitted boats it is a convenient method of finding position.

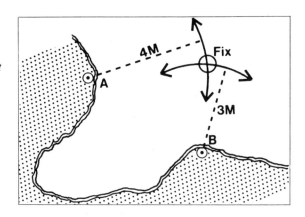

Fig. 106 *Light A, range 4 miles. Light B, range 3 miles*

Using the sextant

With the instrument set at 0°, the view through the telescope would be as in Fig. 107a. A vertical sextant angle is taken by winding the image seen in the mirror down, until the light is touching the shoreline seen through the clear glass, as in Fig. 107b. The reading on the sextant corrected for any index error is the VSA. To find the angle between two shore marks, the instrument is turned through 90° so that the frame is parallel to the ground. The right hand object of the two is viewed in the mirror — again with the sextant set at 0° — and its image is moved left until it superimposes with the other fixing mark as in Fig. 108. The reading on the sextant is the HSA. Index error may be ignored.

Fig. 107a *VSA. Sextant set at 0° b When the shoreline bisects the light, the VSA is read off*

Fig. 108 *HSA. The right hand mark is moved left until the two marks superimpose*

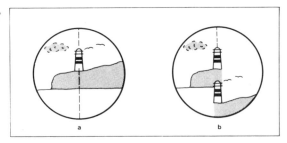

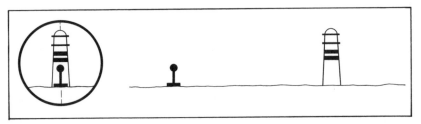

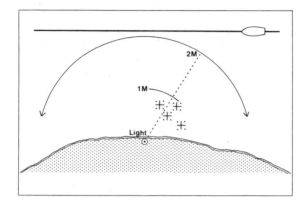

Fig. 109 *Danger angle. Use of VSA to stay at least 2 miles from the light, thus clearing the rocks by a mile*

Danger angle

When only one charted lighthouse is visible, a vertical sextant angle can be used to ensure that a vessel is safe. Fig. 109 shows a boat that wants to pass 2 miles off the light, giving a safety margin of 1 mile from the rocks. The VSA is found by entering the tables with the height of and required distance from the light. This *danger angle*, as it is called, is set on the sextant. As long a there is a gap between the top of the light seen in the mirror and the shoreline below it seen through the clear glass, the vessel is in safe water.

Although the light may be clearly visible, it may not be possible to see the shoreline beneath from a small boat because of the earth's curvature. Thus distance by VSA may not be accurate at much over 3 miles. Another limitation is that the lighthouse must be right on the coastline. Any buildings set in land must not be used when finding distances by VSA. Charted heights are given above the level of mean high water springs, and as the tide falls the height of the light increases. Allowance must be made for the height of the tide for fully accurate results. However, the error caused by using the charted height at half or low tide errs on the safe side. The distance off from the table is less than the true distance, the boat would appear closer to the coast than it was in reality and any avoiding action would be taken sooner than strictly necessary.

Chapter Eight
Winds and Weather

The term 'weather' describes the state of the atmosphere at any given time and place. The state of the atmosphere determines the winds and the strength of the winds controls the sea conditions. Any seafarer has a vital interest in the weather — the amateur boat owner more so in some ways than the big ship man because the winds and seas experienced on the coast can be just as damaging to a small craft as any midwinter north Atlantic galé to an ocean-going vessel.

While the reader may not need to go into the subject in as much depth as the professionals, an outline knowledge will allow him to make reasonable short-term weather predictions. Secondly, an understanding of the jargon used in the newspaper or on the radio will give added meaning in interpreting official forecasts. Navigation is the art of getting a boat *safely* from A to B, and meteorology is part and parcel of the same subject.

Meteorology is a comparatively recent science because it cannot function without a widespread, fast and reliable communication system. Certain facts such as pressure, temperature, wind directions and cloud formations must be collected from various places so that the weather picture over a country or ocean can be drawn up and a forecast made on the basis of this information.

The Meteorological Office was established in London in 1854, and other national weather bureaux came into being in Europe at about the same time. The first telegraphic weather report, however, appeared in the *London Daily News* on 31 August 1848, and with the spread of the telegraph, meteorology soon became a worldwide science. Meteorological observations began in Australia at Parramatta as early as 1822, and were in full swing at the Sydney Observatory by 1859. The daily construction of weather maps was started in the 1870s by the Government Astronomer. In New Zealand, the first ten permanent stations were approved by the government in 1859. The first public weather forecasts and a storm warning organisation for shipping were begun in 1874. I have no knowledge of the accuracy of the predictions they made, but modern meteorologists insist that a forecast is only *the most likely* of a number of possible outcomes in the future weather, based on the information available at the time.

Air and the atmosphere

The envelope of air surrounding the earth is called the atmosphere, and consists of a mixture of gases, mostly nitrogen and oxygen. The air also contains water vapour in varying amounts, found mainly in the first 10 000 m. The total water vapour in a given mass of air depends entirely on the temperature. The hotter the air, the more vapour it can hold.

The atmosphere is divided into a number of layers, only two of which directly concern the weather. The lower one, called the *troposphere*, reaches in height from ground level to about 5 miles above the poles, increasing to 11 miles over the equator. The majority of all weather takes place in the troposphere, and usually the higher one goes, the colder it gets. The next layer, reaching to about 30 miles, is the *stratosphere*. Here the temperature reverses its previous trend and increases with height, giving a more stable atmosphere than in the weather-torn troposphere below it.

Wind flow

Wind is a movement or flow of air from one place to another and is described by the direction from which it comes. The earlier mariners spoke of 'the wind blowing from the south'. As this phrase was a bit of a mouthful it was inevitably shortened to 'a south wind'.

To understand the general flow of air in the atmosphere, let us first consider a non-rotating earth. The tropics are hotter than the polar regions. Warm air around the equator would rise and be replaced by cooler, heavier air from the temperate zones. This air would in turn be replaced by cold, dense air from each of the poles. The warm, light equatorial air in the upper atmosphere would flow towards the poles in each hemisphere, cooling as it went. The further it moved from the equator, the colder and heavier it would become, finally sinking back to earth in the two polar regions and replacing the cold air at the surface which was starting its journey to the tropics. If the earth did not rotate, there would be a simple pattern of surface winds blowing directly north or south from each pole to the equator, due to the cycle of warming and cooling described above.

However, the spin of the earth from west to east deflects the winds away from their strictly north-south directions. As the surface flow of air moves from the North Pole towards the equator it curves to the right, changing the north wind into a north-easterly and then an easterly wind. In the Southern Hemisphere the curve is to the left as air flows from the South Pole and the wind direction changes from south to south-east and then again east. This would still give a simple cycle of upper air moving to each of the poles and a surface wind flow back to the equator.

120

In practice, the general flow of air around the earth is divided into a number of east-west bands, each with a fairly well defined pattern of winds. Even so, within each wind belt local weather systems build up and die away again, giving us the ever-changing pattern we call the weather. Air has weight and exerts a pressure. Naturally at ground level the more air there is over a given part of the earth's surface or the colder and therefore denser the air, the heavier it will be. By comparison with lighter air at some neighbouring part of the earth, it will have a higher pressure. Each of the wind belts straddling the earth has a different average pressure than the adjoining belt. Thus one would be said to have either a higher or lower pressure than its neighbours, but this is not to be confused with the self-contained high and low pressure systems confined to a particular ocean or locality that are described later.

As already explained, the general movement of air starts with an upper wind flow away from the equator towards each pole. These upper air flows are also deflected due to the spin of the earth, and by the time they reach latitudes 30° north and south, most of this flow has become westerly. This causes a build-up of air in the regions of 30° latitude, giving a higher pressure belt than in the tropics where the air is rising. Much of this air subsides and this gives the clear skies and warm temperatures associated with the anticyclones of the high pressure belt. At ground level some of the air moves back towards the lower pressure tropics. In the Northern Hemisphere it curves to the right due to the twist imparted by the earth's spin, giving the north-east trade winds, and in the Southern Hemisphere it curves to the left, giving the south-east trades. The remainder of the descending air continues its flow back towards each pole and, on being deflected, gives the prevailing surface westerlies that blow over the middle latitudes in both hemispheres. The remaining high level air moves on towards the poles, cooling as it goes. Finally cold heavy air sinks down to the surface at each of the polar regions, giving areas of relatively higher pressure than in the adjoining belts of the prevailing westerlies. The subsequent surface winds blowing from the poles towards the equator curve right (Northern Hemisphere) and left (Southern Hemisphere) to give the polar easterlies.

The boundary lines between the cold polar air and the relatively warmer surface air in the two belts of westerlies are called the polar fronts. The word *front* is used to describe the line at which any large mass of warm air meets a mass of cold air. There is no sharply defined line between the two as shown in weather maps. Each polar front may have bends and curves in it, and the ground-hugging dense cold air may push under the warmer air, forcing it up. The rising warm air cools rapidly, giving turbulent conditions, and much of the bad weather we experience is generated at the polar fronts.

Nothing is certain in the weather world, but some general characteristics apply to each of the wind zones.

Beaufort	Description	Knots	Sea conditions	Sailing conditions for cruising keelboats
0	Calm	<1	Sea like a mirror.	No headway and sails slatting.
1	Light air	1–3	Scale-like ripples form but without foam crests.	Good steerage way to boats before the wind
2	Light breeze	4–6	Small wavelets, still short but more pronounced. Crests have a glassy appearance but do not break.	Boats on the wind moving well. Spinnakers fill.
3	Gentle breeze	7–10	Large wavelets; crests begin to break; foam of glassy appearance; perhaps scattered white horses.	Good way on all boats which begin to heel. Spinnakers filled and lifting.
4	Moderate breeze	11–16	Small waves, becoming longer; fairly frequent white horses.	Good working breeze for all craft. Yachts on the wind well heeled over. Optimum conditions for large genoas.
5	Fresh breeze	17–21	Moderate waves taking a more pronounced long form; many white horses are formed (chance of some spray).	Boats reach designed hull speed. Spinnakers marginal, but large genoas at limit.
6	Strong breeze	22–27	Large waves begin to form. White foam crests are more extensive everywhere. Some spray.	Reefing recommended for cruising craft.
7	Near gale (moderate gale – USA)	28–33	Sea heaps up and white foam from breaking waves begins to be blown in streaks along the direction of the wind.	Reefing a must for cruising craft and most will be seeking shelter.

8	Gale (fresh gale)	34–40	Moderately high waves of greater length; edges of crests begin to break into spindrift; foam is blown in well-marked streaks along the direction of the wind.	Storm foresail weather with main double-reefed or possibly trysail if it can still be carried. Go home.
9	Strong gale	41–47	High waves; dense streaks of foam along the direction of the wind. Wave tops tumble and spray may affect visibility.	Too late. Heave to or make for deep water clear of land. Possibly bare-pole sailing at upper limit of wind speed with warps streamed.
10	Storm (whole gale)	48–55	Very high waves with long overhanging crests. The surface of the sea takes on a white appearance and foam in great patches is blown in dense white streaks along the direction of the wind. The tumbling of the sea becomes heavy and shocklike; visibility affected.	Wind and sea limit for most cruising boats which will be forced to scud or stream sea anchors.
11	Violent storm (storm) and	56–63	Exceptionally high waves, air is filled with foam and spray; sea completely white with driving spray; visibility very seriously affected and other vessels lost to view behind waves.	No data.
12	Hurricane	64 and over		

Fig. 110 *The Beaufort wind scale*

123

The *westerlies* are the major air flow between about latitudes 30° and 60°. They are far from permanent, being interspersed by areas of bad weather moving from west to east; the winds can vary greatly in both strength and direction. The continental land masses in the Northern Hemisphere with their mountain ranges and other topographical features also break up the wind flow. However, in the southern oceans the winds can blow unimpeded across thousands of miles of open sea. Westerly winds, often of great force, blow more constantly and the area around latitude 40°S was called the *roaring forties* by the sailing ship captains.

The *variables* straddle the latitudes of 30° in each hemisphere. In this higher pressure belt where the air is sinking, the winds are weak and unreliable. The air is warmed by the compression from the weight of air above and there is no transfer of heat as there is at the polar front, so skies tend to be cloudless. These are called the *horse latitudes* in the Northern Hemisphere. The term is thought to have originated when ships carrying horses as cargo from Europe to the Americas were becalmed for long periods.

Critical water shortages resulted and the horses, dead or dying of thirst, were tossed overboard. Other ships reported that at times the sea was littered with the bodies of the animals.

The *trade winds* blow on either side of the equator. The north-east trade wind blows with great persistence, averaging about 15 knots, although this can vary with the season and in different oceans. The south-east trade is not as reliable and on average the wind strength is a little less. The weather in the trade wind zones is generally fair with only small amounts of cloud.

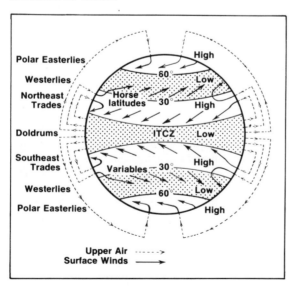

Fig. 111 *The earth: wind and pressure belts*

The *doldrums* occur in the lower pressure area around the equator between the trade wind belts. The name was given by sailing ship men who could find themselves becalmed for lack of wind for days or weeks on end. Despite the region's notoriety for lack of wind, there can be marked variations in the conditions experienced. Mariners find oppressively hot, windless weather can change with little warning to vicious squalls, torrential rain and thunderstorms.

Wind strength

Wind speeds are usually given in knots these days, but a scale devised by Admiral Sir Francis Beaufort of the Royal Navy in 1808 is still used in many quarters. The wind strength is described by a number from 0 (calm) to 12 (hurricane force) and is shown in Fig. 110. These are mean wind speeds, in the open sea, and there may be occasional much stronger gusts. For a given wind speed the waves may be much shorter and steeper in coastal waters than those described in the table for the open sea.

The admiral described Force 1 as being just sufficient to 'give steering way to a full-rigged ship' and so on up to Force 12 when 'no canvas can stand'. These descriptions were later adapted for 'your average-sized sailing trawler', but as neither of these is much use to the yachtsman, the table has been adjusted accordingly.

By using the wind speeds given in the radio weather forecast, the yachtsman can see from Fig. 110 what the sailing conditions are likely to be on any particular day.

Local winds

Many types of local wind are found in various parts of the world but the most widely spread and most useful to the yachtsman are the land and sea breezes. They occur all year round in the tropics and are found around coastlines situated in more temperate climates during the summer and early autumn. These winds alternate between a breeze swinging off the land at night and a wind blowing in from the sea by day.

Sea breeze

The sea breeze blows from seaward towards the land, starting in the late morning and reaching maximum strength two to three hours after noon. During the day the land heats more quickly than the sea; air in contact with the land is heated by conduction and radiation and rises. The thermal updraughts are replaced by cooler air moving in from the sea. The continuing cycle results in a steady onshore wind that dies away at about sunset. The 'Fremantle Doctor' is an excellent example of a sea breeze that gained world wide fame, or notoriety, during the 1986/87 Americas Cup.

Land breeze

The land breeze is an offshore wind that sets in during the night, although

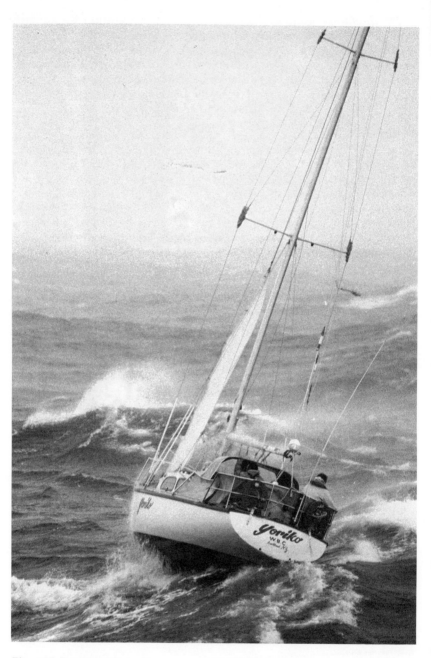

Fig. 112 *Beaufort Force 8*

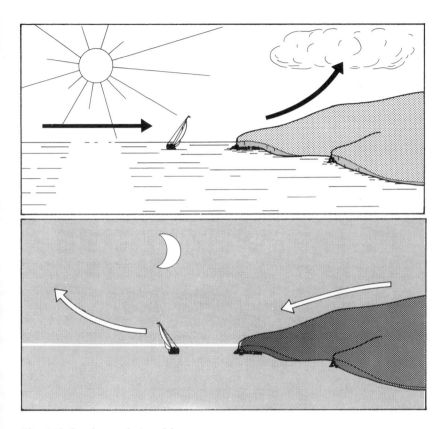

Fig. 113 *Sea breeze* b *Land breeze*

it is not as reliable or as strong as the daytime sea breeze. It is caused by a reversal in the unequal heating of land and sea. After sunset the land cools quickly, especially if a clear sky allows rapid radiation of heat into the atmosphere. The heat loss from the sea is at a much slower rate. The warmer air over the sea rises and cold air flows off the land to replace it. If there is a steep coast with higher ground behind, the process is assisted by the colder, heavier air flowing seaward down the slope due to the influence of gravity.

Katabatic winds are another type of offshore wind caused by cold, dense air draining from high ground. Where the coast is backed by snow-covered mountains, very cold air accumulates around the peaks. Even a light offshore wind is enough to start this air literally falling down the mountain valleys, gathering speed as it goes. It can reach the coast without warning as a strong or even gale force wind, and can be a danger to small boats at anchor or sailing in what had previously been light, pleasant winds.

The importance of heat

The astronauts have confirmed that there is neither an atmosphere nor weather on the moon. We also know that there is no weather in our stratosphere. If there was no water vapour in the troposphere, no rain would fall.

Air will flow from an area of higher pressure to an area of lower pressure causing a wind. The ingredients necessary to cause weather, or more correctly weather changes, seem to be an atmosphere, water vapour and air pressure differences or wind. While this is correct as far as it goes, the fundamental energy source necessary in creating weather is *heat*.

The prime source of heat is the sun. Energy from the sun reaches the earth in the form of short-wave radiations including, of course, light waves. There are also ultra-violet and infra-red rays which cannot be seen by the human eye. Although these are not heat waves, they change to heat when absorbed by more solid objects such as the earth's crust or the oceans. About 43 per cent of the total incoming solar energy passes through the atmosphere to the earth's surface, heats what it touches and is re-radiated as heat energy.

In the process, an important change takes place. The earth-radiated heat has a longer wavelength than the incoming solar energy and is too long to escape readily through the atmosphere back into space. Much of this radiant heat from the earth is absorbed by water vapour in the air. The water vapour results from evaporation due to the heating of the oceans and lakes. Thus, like a greenhouse, the atmosphere lets in the sun's short-wave radiations and traps most of the outgoing heat waves, acting as a thermal insulator. However, this heat is distributed in a very random fashion. The sun's rays rebound back into the atmosphere from highly reflective surfaces such as the polar ice caps without the intermediate steps of absorption and change to radiant heat. Bare rock or barren land areas on the earth absorb most of the sun's rays, becoming very hot in the process and then releasing much of this radiant heat back into the atmosphere. On a global scale, the summertime half of the earth will release far more energy than the other with its colder winter temperatures. This highly uneven distribution of heat sets the weather process in motion. Thus the underlying cause of all weather is not heat itself, but the transfer of heat from one part of the world to another, or from one air mass to another, whenever and wherever they meet and mix.

The combination of the effect of the earth's rotation and unequal surface heating leads to the formation of self-contained weather systems within the more general wind zones circling the earth. These may consist of good weather high-pressure cells called highs or anti-cyclones, or bad weather low-pressure systems called lows, depressions or cyclones. These weather systems vary in size from a few hundred to 1000 or even 2000 miles in diameter. The highest pressure is at the centre of an anti-cyclone and decreases on moving outward from the centre. The lowest pressure is at the centre of a cyclonic system and increases with distance from the centre.

Atmospheric pressure

The atmospheric pressure varies from place to place and from time to time, but a normal value is quite well known.

The metric unit of atmospheric pressure is the hectopascal (hPa), which is 100 pascals. The International Meteorological Organisation decreed that the hPa replace the millibar (mb), which was used until about 1990. As 1mb = 1 hPa, the conversion from one to the other is fairly straightforward. A column of air extending from sea level to the top of the atmosphere exerts the same pressure on the surface of the earth as does a column of mercury 760 mm in height. The standard pressure equivalent to the columns of air or mercury is 1013.25 hPa. An average high may be from 1015 to 1025, and an average low around 990 to 1000 hPa.

Measuring pressure

The instrument used to measure air pressure is the *barometer*.

A mercurial barometer consists of a glass tube almost a metre in height, sealed at one end, open at the other and filled with mercury. The column of mercury rises and falls depending on the pressure on the open end, and the pressure is read off on a scale graduated in millibars. It is by

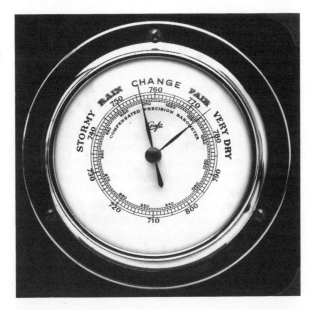

Fig. 114 *An aneroid barometer*

far the most accurate barometer but is bulky, expensive and fragile.

The compact aneroid barometer is a little less accurate, but being less expensive and more robust it is ideal for small boats. Basically it consists of a corrugated sealed metal container. The air is removed, forming a vacuum, and the corrugations plus an internal spring prevent the outside air pressure from collapsing the chamber. However, the top of the container bows in or out with increases or decreases in atmospheric pressure. These movements are transmitted by gears and levers to a pointer on a dial. Barometers graduated in millibars will be quite common for a decade or so.

CLOUDS

There is always water in the atmosphere due to the constant cycle of evaporation but it is very unevenly distributed around the earth. The amount of water vapour in the air at a given locality is called the *humidity*.

When the amount of water vapour in the air is expressed as a percentage of the total that could be held at the particular temperature, it is called the *relative humidity*.

When air rises, it is cooled as it ascends for two reasons. Firstly, in the troposphere temperature decreases with height; secondly, the surrounding pressure decreases as it rises and the air expands. Expansion is a cooling process. If the air rises high enough, the relative humidity reaches 100 per cent and on further rising and cooling, water vapour condenses out in the form of droplets forming clouds. If the droplets merge with one another there comes a stage where they are too heavy to remain aloft and it rains. Most clouds are in the troposphere but some have great vertical development and jut into the lower stratosphere. The tops of these clouds usually consist of ice crystals, and most high clouds are entirely made up of ice crystals.

Cloud names

Clouds are classified according to how they are formed and there are two basic types. The first type, caused by rising air currents, is puffy or piled-up and known as *cumulus clouds*. The second type of cloud is formed when a layer of air is cooled below the water vapour saturation point without upwards movement. These layered formations are called *stratus clouds*. The word *fracto* is added to describe wind-blown clouds that have been broken into pieces. *Nimbus*, meaning 'rain', is added to the names of clouds which characteristically bring rain or snow. As the same basic formation clouds can be found at varying heights, their altitude is indicated by using the words *alto*, meaning 'middle', and *cirrus*, indicating very high clouds composed almost wholly of ice crystals.

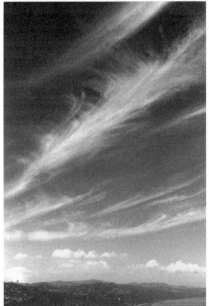

Fig. 115 *Cirrus*

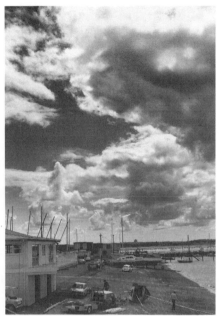

Fig. 116 *Stratocumulus*

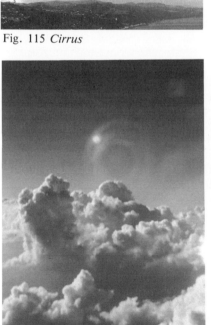

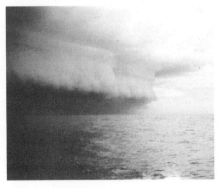

Fig. 118 *Squall line roll cloud.*

Fig. 117 *Bird's eye view of cumulus with vertical development*

131

Cloud types

Cirrus (Ci) clouds are usually seen first in the high western sky forming delicate filaments, patches or narrow bands. Those shaped like commas and often called mare's tails, indicate that a warm front is approaching.

Cirrostratus (Cs) are high layered clouds, transparent enough to let the sun shine through. The ice crystals in these can cause the large halos sometimes seen around the sun or moon. They usually indicate approaching rain.

Cirrocumulus (Cc) are thin, white clouds, rippled or in layers with some vertical development in the form of turrets. When these clouds appear uniformly in ripples they give what seamen call a mackerel sky. They are usually too thin to cast shadows and indicate a continuing period of fair weather (except on those days when rain follows). If the reader thinks that this description is not particularly helpful, blame the weather, not the writer. There is a saying in my neck of the woods that goes, 'If you think the weather's good, wait a minute.'

Altostratus (As) clouds are greyish, layered or fibrous clouds that cover most of the sky. These clouds are fairly reliable indicators of approaching rain or the development of stormy conditions at sea.

Altocumulus (Ac) usually occur as extensive sheets of white and grey cloudlets with a rounded appearance. They are a good indication of impending rain.

Nimbostratus (Ns) clouds are the rain carriers. Low, uniform in appearance and dark, they cannot be mistaken for anything other than rain clouds. They are useless for forecasting because the bad weather has already arrived. However, there may still be time to seek shelter from the accompanying high wind and resulting seas.

Stratus (St) are low, grey layered clouds, giving the sky a leaden look. Their appearance will almost certainly mean light rain or drizzle, but there is little danger from high winds.

Stratocumulus (Sc) are low, irregular layers of white or grey clouds accompanied by dark patches in the shape of rounded masses or rolls. They give dull but probably clearing conditions with rain unlikely.

Cumulus (Cu) clouds are the cotton-wool fluffy ones with constantly changing shapes. When detached with only slight vertical development they are aptly termed 'fair weather cumulus'. However, when cumulus clouds start to tower into the sky in great rolls, they are likely to bring gusty surface winds and heavy showers.

Cumulonimbus (Cb) are heavy, dense clouds with massive vertical development, sometimes with flattened tops in the shape of an anvil. These are the thunderheads, bringing heavy rain, lightning and frequently hail.

PRESSURE AND WIND

Pressure readings received at national weather centres from a myriad of reporting stations, including ships at sea, are plotted on a large map. All this information forms the basis for the daily weather forecasts and simplified weather maps seen on television or in the daily newspapers.

On these maps, the lines joining all points with the same pressure are called *isobars*. These are equivalent to contour lines on maps, and the density or distance apart of the isobars indicates the wind strength. The isobars around the fair weather high-pressure systems are generally widely spaced, while those around the foul weather lows are much closer together. Contour lines on maps show the gradient or steepness of high ground or hills. Meteorologists refer to the distance apart of the isobars as the *pressure gradient*.

If the earth were not spinning, the wind would blow in a direction at right angles across the isobars from a higher to a lower pressure. But the earth does spin and there is also a slowing effect on the lower winds due to friction between the earth's surface and the moving air in contact with it. the result of these two factors is that surface winds blow around

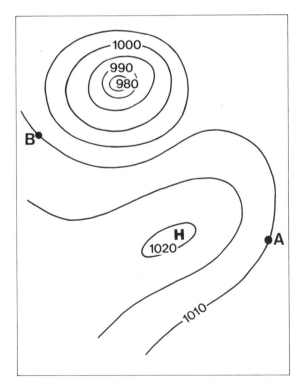

Fig. 119 *Isobars around high and low pressure areas*

the centre of an anti-cyclone or a depression almost parallel to the isobars. However, at and near ground level in ocean areas, the wind spirals out of high pressure regions into low pressure ones in a direction that crosses the isobars at an angle of about 15°. Over land areas that give greater friction, this angle increases to about 30°.

Any fluid moving across a stationary surface is itself at rest where the two are in contact, due to drag. So when air blows across a denser surface such as earth or water it is virtually stopped where the two meet. However, its mean speed increases with distance or height above ground or sea level as the drag lessens, until an unretarded free stream is reached. This increase or decrease in mean wind speed with gain or loss of height is loosely termed wind shear.

The free speed of the surface wind is at an altitude of about 600 metres, but successive layers of are air moving at different speeds. Strictly speaking the shear is the difference in mean wind speed between any two layers. The surface wind over land is about one third of the 600-metre wind and over the open sea is about two thirds. So if the mean speed at 600 metres was 30 knots, the wind at sea level is likely to be 20 knots, and the shear is 10 knots. Forecast surface winds are for a height of 10 metres, so a boat's anemometer at say, 5 metres may register a lower mean wind speed, the difference being the (vertical) shear.

When the free speed exceeds a certain limit the flow breaks down into a turbulent motion and the friction layer with the earth or sea becomes much deeper. This turbulence set up by surface drag can cause quite marked changes in the atmosphere.

From the yachtsman's point of view the wind speed can more than double in the first 30 metres. This did not matter too much with older cruising boats, but for present day maxis and the larger family yachts it becomes a factor to consider when deciding what sails to hoist, or whether there should be another reef in the main.

Take, for example, a boat where the sail is about 15 metres from top to bottom. If the surface wind was 8 knots, it might increase to ten at the foot of the sail, and then to 16 knots at the head.

Pressure systems
Highs
In general these are the fine weather systems and, certainly near the centre, they are characterised by clear skies, light to moderate winds with calm seas and perhaps a long, low ocean swell. However, fog can form near the centre or on the outer edges when warm air moves over cold water.

The wind circulation around a high is clockwise in the Northern Hemisphere, anti-clockwise in the Southern Hemisphere.

They generally move eastward at about 15 knots, but are often stationary for long periods. The temperatures can be either warm or cold with little or no change for relatively long periods.

Lows
These inevitably mean impending bad weather to a greater or lesser degree. The lower or deeper the central pressure, the stronger will be the associated winds. These depressions are characterised by a variety of cloud types, bringing moderate to heavy rain and sometimes snow. The strong winds may shift abruptly, turning what will already be large waves into confused omnidirectional seas. Stormy conditions generally result.

Fig 119 shows a high-pressure system and a depression as they appear on a weather map. Notice that the isobars around the high are quite widely spaced, indicating light winds, while those around the low are much closer together. Between the centre of the high and the point A — a distance of 500 miles — the pressure only changes from 1020 to 1010, or 10 millibars. On the other hand, between point B and the centre of the low, which is also 500 miles, the pressure changes by 25 millibars. The greater the change in pressure over the same distance, the stronger the winds will be.

The wind blows anti-clockwise around a depression in the Northern Hemisphere and clockwise in the Southern Hemisphere. Like the highs, they move from west to east, but average 18 knots, rising to 25 knots in the winter months. They can also become stationary. Air temperatures are usually cold but can be warm at first, changing to cold. The direction of the centre of the depression can be estimated by facing directly into the wind and the centre of low pressure then lies 112° on the right hand in north latitudes, on the left hand in south latitudes.

When highs become higher and lows lower, the correct expressions to use are 'a high intensifying' or 'a deepening depression'. If the reverse is happening the low is said to be *filling* and the high *weakening*.

Trough of low pressure
Occasionally an area of low pressure may appear on the weather chart as a long slender shape reaching between two anti-cyclones. This pressure formation jutting into the higher pressure area is called a *trough of low pressure* and has weather similar to a weak cold front (see page 147).

Ridge of high pressure
Sometimes an elongated band of high pressure is found between two depressions or troughs of low pressure. A brief period of fine weather may be experienced in this narrow band which is called a ridge of high pressure.

Air streams
This country is surrounded by sea, and air blowing from either the tropics or the pole is called Maritime air. It is moist in both cases, but Tropical

135

Maritime air is warm and moist while Polar Maritime air is cool and moist. These two air streams play a significant part in our weather. By the way, when a meteorologist says warm, he means hot, and if he says cool then turn the heaters up. If they actually say cold during the winter, then its brass monkey weather.

Out at sea, Tropical Maritime air will bring warm weather with layer cloud and possibly light rain. Polar Maritime air means colder weather with showers from cumulus type clouds, but otherwise good visibility. Closer to the coast the weather from either air mass should be much the same as found at sea, but over land there can be quite different conditions experienced on the windward and leeward coasts.

Where the windward coast is backed by high hills or a mountain range, the moist air will be forced to rise, become colder forming cloud and will then lose most of its moisture as rain. It then descends on the lee side as drier warmer air and blows across country giving fine stable conditions on the leeward coast. A good example of this is when a westerly airstream is forced to rise over the Southern Alps, dumping its rain on the West Coast and blowing across the plains to arrive at the east or leeward coast as a hot dry wind giving good weather. This is called a fohn wind.

Diurnal variations
There is a regular daily or diurnal change in pressure of about 2 mbs in temperate latitudes, increasing to about 3 mbs in the tropics. Maximum pressure occurs at 1000 and 2200, and the minimum at 0400 and 1600. This effect is often masked by greater changes due to an approaching high or low pressure system.

These daily pressure changes cause a diurnal change in mean wind speed of about 2 knots in temperate latitudes, with the minimum at 0900 and maximum at 1500. Again this diurnal variation can be masked by much greater changes in wind speed due to the prevailing pressure system.

Frontal systems
As mentioned earlier, a front is the boundary or meeting of two different air masses and on a global scale there are several that are more or less permanent. Of these the most important are the polar fronts in both hemispheres, separating cold polar air from the warmer temperate zone air masses. The Mediterranean front separates the cold winter air over Europe from the warm air over North Africa. The Intertropical Convergence Zone (ITCZ), once known as the Intertropical or Equatorial Front, is the belt separating the north-east and south-east trade winds on each side of the equator. While not a true front, because temperature and moisture conditions in the atmosphere on either side of the ITCZ are much the same, it is the breeding zone for many of the highly destructive tropical revolving storms.

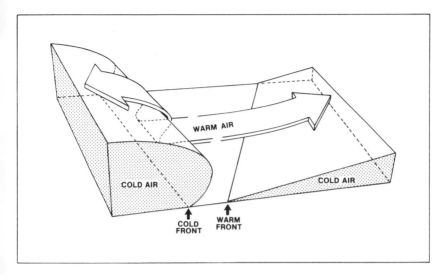

COLD AIR

COLD AIR

WARM AIR

COLD
FRONT

WARM
FRONT

Fig. 120 *Fronts*

However, to the temperate zone yachtsman, the word front is usually associated with the more localised atmospheric disturbances which are shown as a line on a weather map and bring with them all those changes in the weather.

This line can be misleading because two dissimilar air masses, one possibly cold and dry and the other warm and moist, are not rectangular blocks placed side by side like two bricks, i.e., the front does not extend vertically straight up from ground level. It is impossible to show the shape of a front between say 0 and 6000 metres on a weather map, so in this context the front is the line at the *earth's surface* at which cold and warm air meet. Remember that, regardless of the type of front, there is cold air on one side of it and warm air on the other.

Despite this meteorologists insist on calling one type a warm and the other a cold front. Briefly, a cold front occurs if cold air is advancing, and a warm front if warm air is advancing. They are always associated with a low or depression and usually move to the eastward, but can become stationary. One can occur without the other, but where they are associated with the same depression, the warm front arrives first, followed by the faster-moving cold front. If the latter overtakes and merges with the warm front they are said to be *occluded*.

Warm fronts
Here warm air advances, replacing cold air at the earth's surface. However, ground friction slows up the bottom edge of the retreating cold air and the fast-moving warm air is forced up over the cold, giving the sloping frontal surface shown in Fig. 120. The warm front weather

137

can extend hundreds of miles in advance of the line of the front at ground level. The rising warm air cools, forming cloud, and the cloud type depends on its height up the slope. The first sign of an approaching warm front is high cirrus cloud in the western sky which gradually lowers to cirrostratus. The barometer begins to fall and as the cloud base lowers still further, giving altocumulus and altostratus, rain begins to fall and continues until the front has passed. When the front is weak the cloud formation will be much less marked with perhaps only light rain or drizzle. The temperature will rise with the passage of the front and the barometer will level off.

The frontal slope is relatively gentle and, although the warm air rises, there is only a slow progressive cooling which leads to an orderly formation of cloud. There may be little change in the direction of the wind as the front passes, but if there is, it will veer in the Northern Hemisphere and back in the Southern Hemisphere.

Cold fronts

The fast-moving cold front that follows is so called because cold air is replacing warm air at the frontal surface. Friction between the ground and the lower air tends to hold back the bottom of the advancing cold air mass and the higher, faster-moving air curls over ahead of the ground-level frontal line, forming a wedge. The cold air, in forging its way ahead, makes the warm air rise abruptly with consequent rapid cooling leading to heavy cloud formation over the front, but it has no great depth. Thus the storms brought by cold fronts are usually violent but relatively brief. If the air ahead of the front is particularly hot and very humid, it will be forced so high so quickly that cumulonimbus thunderheads will form,

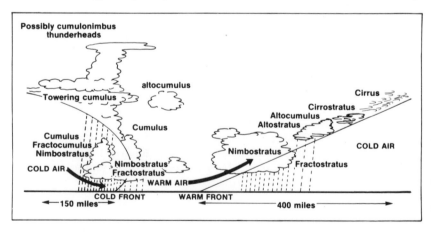

Fig. 121 *Cloud types associated with the passing of* a *a warm and* b *a cold front*

giving heavy thunder showers in addition to the rain from the lower nimbostratus.

The approach of the front is heralded by a falling barometer with lowering clouds in the western sky and a darkening horizon. Heavy rain falls with the approach of cumulonimbus clouds and may quickly increase in intensity, as will the wind strength as the barometer continues falling. When the front passes, the wind shifts rapidly in direction by up to 90° with strong gusts and it is noticeably colder. Squally weather continues with the barometer reaching its lowest point. Once the front has passed the cloud and rain usually clear swiftly and the barometer rises rapidly. With any luck, there should be a few days of good weather following until another approaching group of cirrus high in the western sky shows that the whole cycle of warm and cold front weather is about to start again.

Line squalls
Fast moving cold fronts are frequently preceded by line squalls, so called because they appear as a roll of black cloud often stretching right across the sky. When the line squall hits, the wind shifts with almost explosive violence and torrential rain falls behind the leading edge.

Cold front waves
Most cold fronts that cross this country are associated with depressions that form south of Tasmania and then move east to pass south of New Zealand. However, some depressions can form in mid-Tasman on an existing cold front when, for whatever reason, there is a lowering of pressure at one point on the front and a new cyclonic circulation develops. These cold front wave depressions or secondaries tend to move south and can often absorb the primary depression, but in turn another wave depression can form on the cold front associated with the secondary. There can be up to three of these lows at the one time, and on a weather map the connecting cold fronts look like a series of waves running roughly north/south. A secondary low can be very active, but the weather experienced as it passes through is the same as for any depression and cold front system.

Sea and swell waves
To the mariner, waves can range in size from those lapping on the gentle shore to the ocean monsters that stand above a tall ship's mast as it plunges in the trough between. Yet the life cycle of any wave is much the same. It is generated by the wind, grows gradually to a maximum size depending on certain limiting factors, then journeys across the sea and may gradually lose height until it arrives as a swell on some distant coast.

The term swell is given to waves that have been generated at a distance, usually by a storm, or the residual waves in an area when the wind has ceased to blow. 'Sea' is used to describe the waves resulting by a wind blowing in the local area. The succession of waves resulting from a given wind is called a wave train, but where there are both a long distance swell and a local sea running, the two wave trains can combine to give higher seas. If the sea and swell wave trains are running across each other, then the resulting turbulence can give very rough seas even if each wave train is only slight or moderate.

These expressions 'slight', 'moderate', and 'rough' seas when used by the weatherman are more traps for young players. The height of a wave is the vertical distance from trough to crest. The internationally agreed average heights of sea waves are:

Slight   .5 to 1.5 metres
Moderate up to 2.5 metres
Rough   up to 4 metres

As these are average heights, some 'slight' waves could be almost head high to an adult.

The size of a wave depends on the strength of the wind, the length of time for which the wind blows, and the open sea distance over which the wind has travelled before arriving at a given spot. This straight line distance is called the fetch. One reason for seeking shelter on the leeward side of an island is that the fetch is too short to allow the waves to build up.

Regardless of the strength of the wind, and even given an unlimited fetch, the waves formed will be at their maximum height after about 30 hours of constant wind.

Short-range weather forecasting

Long-range weather forecasting is still at best an inexact science and a professional meteorologist's daily forecast can be ruined by localised weather disturbances, as we all know. Even so, the yachtsman can make a good stab at short-range weather forecasting and achieve at least a success rate comparable to that of the professionals. Unlike the weather man who, we suspect, works in an office with closed doors and shuttered windows, the yachtsman has the advantage of being forced outdoors where he can see the cloud patterns and discern subtle changes in wind direction and speed. No matter how much the man on the radio may assure his eager listeners that the prospects for a fine sunny day with only light winds could not be better, the yachtsman in the middle of a sail change with the rain oozing down his back remains singularly unimpressed and just *knows* that the weather is going to be awful.

Forecasting is usually based on what is called the persistence method. The assumption is made that a front moving at 15 knots will continue moving at that speed, that a stationary high will remain stationary or that a fast-moving depression heading east will continue the movement

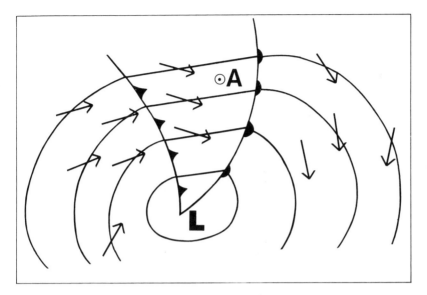

Fig. 122 *Simplified weather map – southern hemisphere*

at the same speed, and so on.

The catch, of course, is that to do any forecasting one needs a weather map. In harbour, those available in the newspapers or elsewhere come complete with a forecast. At sea they can be drawn up by hand, using coded information received by radio, or instant maps are available to larger vessels with weather facsimile receivers. The meteorological people produce excellent brochures explaining the method of using the coded groups to draw the weather picture.

Assuming that the reader has a map, a reasonable forecast can be made for the following six to twelve hours. Fig. 122 shows a simplified weather map giving the situation at 0900. The boat at A is 140 miles ahead of a cold front advancing to the east at 20 knots. The depression is also moving east at 15 knots. At this speed the front will reach A at 1600. The forecast based on these facts and the information already given in this chapter would be:

Situation   A depression to the south is moving away to the east. The associated cold front will reach A late this afternoon.

Forecast   Fine at first, with cloud increasing and scattered showers by late morning. Rain or heavy showers this afternoon. Winds west to north-west, backing south-west and freshening in the afternoon with the passage of the front. Seas slight to moderate. Temperatures moderate at first but cooler tonight and tomorrow.

Further outlook   Clearing weather with some light showers and southerly winds. Seas slight.

Weather lore

Some of the traditional rhymes for forecasting the weather have some scientific basis. Probably the most accurate is:

Red sky at night, sailor's delight,
Red sky in the morning, sailor's warning.

Here the rays of the setting sun light up the high clouds of a cold front that has gone through, and good weather should be on the way. If a front is approaching from the west, then the rays of the rising sun shine on the associated high cloud giving warning of the coming bad weather.

With an approaching depression, if the gale comes first then the following rain seems to flatten the sea. If there is little wind when the rain starts, it will probably blow hard before long. This was recognised in the saying dating back to the days of sail:

When the rain's before the wind,
Topsail halliards you must mind;
When the wind's before the rain,
Hoist your topsails up again.

Other natural signs and their possible meanings include:

A ring round the moon could indicate rain the next day followed by squally winds and rising seas.

Streaky white filaments of high cirrus usually show an approaching front which will arrive within 24 hours.

Heavy jutting cumulus with large bases on the horizon in the morning, with an otherwise fine day, could mean late afternoon thunderstorms.

If seagulls stay over land or fly inland, stormy weather will soon arrive.

Mind you, I heard somewhere the easiest way to decide whether or not it is going to rain is to toss a coin. At least you have a fifty per cent chance of being right.

Chapter Nine
Fog and Foul Weather

FOG

In its most simple terms, fog is a cloud the base of which is resting on or very near the earth's surface. Both cloud and fog consist of droplets of water but they are formed in distinctly different ways. Cloud formation is usually due to rising air that expands and cools. Fog results from the cooling of air that remains at ground level.

When air is holding as much water vapour as it can, it is said to be saturated. The temperature at which air will become saturated is called the *dew point*. Once air is saturated and at its dew point, any further cooling results in condensation appearing in the form of fog or low-lying cloud. Fog is therefore likely to occur when there is only a small difference between the air temperature and the dew point and almost certain when there is no difference at all. If the air is then heated it can hold more water vapour, the dew point rises and the fog disappears.

However, the rate at which fog disperses depends on the actual dew point temperature. Hot air can hold more vapour than cold air before reaching saturation point, so, for a given increase in temperature, air that is already hot can hold much more additional water vapour than can cold air warmed by the same amount. This means that more of the sun's heat is needed to dispel fog at 8°C than at 16°C, even though the total liquid content of the fog itself may be the same in both cases. Thus it takes longer for fog to burn off in colder winter air than it does in summer, also because there is less heat from the sun's rays themselves.

Radiation fog
Radiation fog forms mainly in winter over low-lying land on clear nights that give ideal conditions for rapid cooling of the earth by heat radiation. Air in contact with the earth is cooled below its dew point and the moisture condenses out as fog. Moderate to strong winds prevent fog forming, as does completely calm air when the moisture appears as dew or frost, depending on the ground temperature. Light winds of 3 to 4 knots ensure a continuing supply of wet, warmer air coming in contact with the ground to give more and thicker fog. Although radiation fog

143

does not form at sea because there is only a gradual heat loss from ocean waters during the night, it may drift onto coastal areas and blot out shore-based navigation marks. Light winds may also move a blanket of fog from where it forms at the head of a harbour so that by morning the whole harbour is obscured by the muck. Autumn is also a favourable season for this type of fog because the moisture content of the air is still high. Another favourite spot for radiation fog is the centre of an anti-cyclone because skies are normally clear with light winds. Radiation fog usually disperses by mid- to late morning.

Advection or sea fog
Advection fog may form at any time when moist, warm air flows over a cold water surface, and it is the main type of fog found at sea. The warm air gives off heat to the colder water, is chilled to its dew point and fog forms. Unlike radiation fog, sea fog can be found even in winds up to 20 knots and it is usually extensive and persistent. It may be found in any season but is most common in late spring or early summer in regions where a prevailing warm, moist wind blows over a cold ocean current, or where the sea is very much colder than the air in contact with it. For example, the cold California and Labrador currents cause the summer fog banks off California in the Pacific and off the coasts of Newfoundland and the north-east United States in the north Atlantic. The spring and summer fogs found in the south-west approaches to the English Channel are due to the second cause.

In countries such as Australia and New Zealand where the surrounding seas are relatively warm and there is no great difference between sea and air temperatures, advection fog is unusual.

Frontal fog
Fog of limited extent may form ahead of warm fronts and behind cold fronts. If rain falls from warm air above the frontal surface into the colder air beneath, evaporation of the warm raindrops causes the dew point of the lower air to rise until water vapour condenses out as fog. As this type of fog is confined to a narrow belt, it should clear once the front passes through.

Arctic sea smoke
When very cold air with little or no moisture in it flows over a warmer sea surface there is intense evaporation at the surface. The evaporated moisture saturates the cold air near the surface and immediately condenses out again to form fog. Thus, the sea appears to be smoking or steaming. The conditions are often found in arctic waters when bitterly cold air blows off the polar ice-cap over a sea, which, while at no suitable temperature for a swim, is a whole lot warmer than the icy air − hence the name arctic sea smoke. However, the same thing can be seen to a

lesser degree on inland lakes or even in river valleys during the early morning hours in summer. Very cold air draining down slopes or especially off ice-covered mountains, causes columns of mist or steam to rise off the warmer water surface.

TROPICAL REVOLVING STORMS

Hurricane Caribbean and north-west Atlantic
Typhoon China Sea and north-west Pacific
Cyclone or tropical cyclone Indian Ocean and mid- to south-west Pacific

Tropical revolving storms are known by different names in different oceans as listed above, but all are the same type of intense low pressure weather systems that originate a few degrees north or south of the equator. There are several theories about the reasons for their formation but, regardless of which is, or is not, correct, the facts are undisputed. These storms bring the most violent, destructive and dangerous weather known to the mariner with sustained surface winds of 120 to 150 knots that cause mountainous confused seas. Gusts of 200 knots have been recorded, but the maximum wind speeds are not known for the simple reason that the recording instruments have been blasted from their supports and blown away. The associated waves have been variously estimated at up to and over 20 metres in height, but these are not exact measurements because the people concerned have had more pressing problems on their minds at the time. The rainfall is torrential as shown by one typhoon in the Philippines which brought 2235 millimetres (88 inches) of rain in under four days.

Perhaps the worst single marine disaster this century was when the United States Navy Third Fleet was hit by a typhoon in the north-west Pacific in 1944. Three destroyers capsized and sank with severe loss of life and up to a score of other ships received major or minor damage. Although these examples are extreme, any tropical revolving storm should be treated with respect, especially by the yachtsman.

Tropical cyclones are like the depressions that form outside the tropics in that the wind circulation around the low-pressure area is clockwise in the Southern Hemisphere and counter-clockwise in the Northern Hemisphere, but here the similarity ends. There is no replacement of cold air by warm air and vice versa. The core consists entirely of warm moist tropical air and there are no associated fronts. Tropical cyclones cover a smaller area averaging 400 to 500 miles in diameter. Unlike the middle latitude depressions, they move in a general westerly direction and then curve as explained on page 148. They break up quickly when moving inland although they may wreak havoc in the coastal areas on the way past. There is an almost calm area in the centre or eye of the storm, with light winds and blue skies and this shows up on weather maps where the central isobars form almost perfect circles.

Seasons
Tropical revolving storms can form at any time of the year but are very rare during the winter months. The most critical periods are:
Northern Hemisphere — August to late November
Southern Hemisphere — December to April
One reason for their occurrence during the summer months in each hemisphere is thought to be that the heat needed for their generation requires a sea water temperature of at least 27°C, so the storms are found in the south Pacific but not in the colder south Atlantic.

Formation
The twisting effect of the earth's spin is needed to start a circular movement in any mass of air so these storms rarely form at the equator itself because this effect is cancelled out. However, about 5° away from the equator it is possible for the opposing north-east and south-east trade winds to start a circular movement around each other. The inward-spiralling winds push air towards the centre forcing the hot, moist air to rise. This air cools somewhat on rising and water vapour condenses out. This process releases heat which is trapped in the wind spiral, further heating the air, which becomes lighter and rises more rapidly. Lower down, more tropical air moves in to replace the rising air, there is further condensation and more heat is released which is retained in the heat trap. The tropical revolving storm becomes a self-fuelling vortex with the surrounding tropical air rushing in with ever increasing velocity to form a whirlpool of inward-spiralling cloud and violent winds. The continuous and rapid condensation supplies the moisture for torrential rain.

Wind force
In the early stages, when the storm is in the tropics and covers a relatively small area, winds of more than 60 knots may be encountered up to 100 miles from the centre as well as 40-knot winds out to 200 miles from the lowest pressure. As the storm expands and moves into latitudes of 30° to 35°, there may still be winds of over 30 knots up to 400 miles from the centre.

Waves
The waves produced by the very high winds radiate out in all directions from the centre of the storm. However, the highest waves generated tend to travel in the direction of the storm's movement, and slowly change in character to long swells. As they can move up to 1000 miles per day, while the tropical cyclone itself moves an average of 250–300 miles per day in its early stages, these swells can give good warning of an approaching storm.

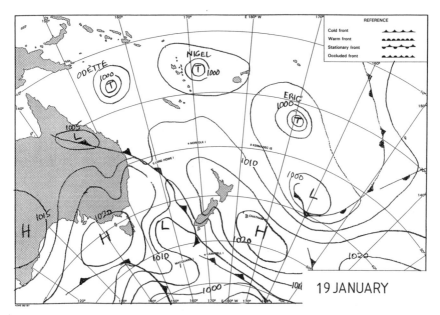

Fig. 123 *Surface weather map showing tropical cyclones Odette, Nigel and Eric. Fiji was hit by Eric on 17 January 1985 with 110 knot winds causing severe damage to houses, crops and coastal craft.*

The eye

The centre of a tropical cyclone is surrounded by a circular wall of cloud, the area of most violent winds and heaviest rain. Visibility is virtually nil due to sheets of almost continuous spray. Inside this ring the winds decrease abruptly to light or moderate and variable, and the rain stops. This feature, unique to tropical storms, is the infamous 'eye', with an average diameter of about 15 miles. It gives a short but deceptive period of relief from the fury of the eye wall. There may be blue sky visible directly overhead but the seas, now coming from all sides may remain heavy or even increase. Across the eye, however, the rain and hurricane-force winds are waiting and will blow from the opposite direction due to the cyclonic circulation. This 180° wind shift has caught many a sailing vessel by surprise, usually to its cost. The eye, of course, being the centre of the storm, is the area of lowest pressure. The barometer can plunge from a reading of about 1000 millibars to less than 900, rising again just as quickly to 980 or so as the centre passes, and then returning to normal over a period of from twelve to eighteen hours.

Tracks

The so-called characteristic tracks followed by tropical revolving storms in each hemisphere are shown in Fig. 125. The cyclone moves off to the west as it forms, at about 10 to 15 knots, and in the later stage of

147

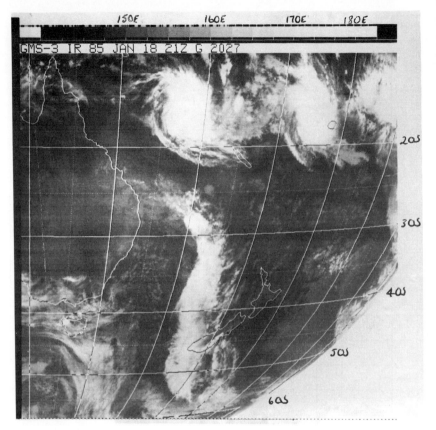

Fig. 124 *GMS weather satellite infra-red photograph taken 6 hours after Fig. 123, showing the tropical storms and the north/south frontal band moving onto New Zealand*

development it curves away from the equator and speeds up. The turn away from the equator continues into higher latitudes where the track recurves so that the storm moves to the north-east in the Northern Hemisphere (south-east in the Southern Hemisphere). After recurving, the storm can move at speeds up to 40 knots although about 25 knots is most common.

One of the biggest problems for the weather man is in forecasting at what stage of its life cycle the recurvature will occur. The other minor problem is that very few tropical cyclones follow the perfect characteristic track. Many storms do not recurve, some move erratically and others become stationary and die out. Once the storm moves out of the hot tropic air it loses its power supply and slowly downgrades to a rain depression although strong winds can persist for some time. They dissipate quickly over continental land masses. Many of the typhoons that hit Hong Kong die out this way by moving on into China; the West

148

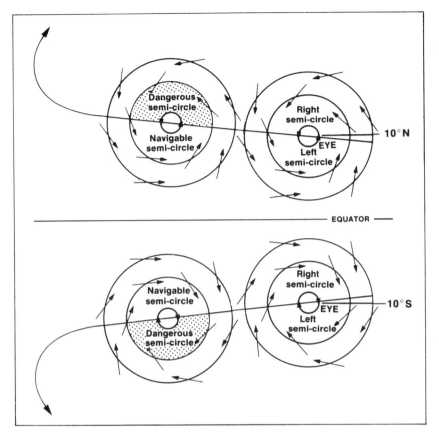

Fig. 125 *Typical tracks of tropical cyclones*: a *Northern Hemisphere*
b *Southern Hemisphere. The left and right semi-circles are on the left and
right hands respectively of an observer on the storm track and facing in the
direction of its movement. This applies to both hemispheres.*

Indian hurricanes also lose intensity after hitting the Florida coast.
However, in the south-west Pacific, the tail end of a cyclone that has
recurved away from the Queensland coast can hammer the north of New
Zealand before filling somewhere to the east of the country.

The worst weather is found in the eye wall but certain parts of the
storm are potentially more dangerous than others. Fig. 126 shows two
boats marked A and B which are ahead of the storm. If boat A were
under reduced sail or forced to heave-to, the southerly winds in south
latitudes would tend to set the boat directly towards the path of the
approaching centre. There is also another danger which depends on the
hemisphere and the boat's tack.

In the Southern Hemisphere a boat close-hauled on the starboard tack

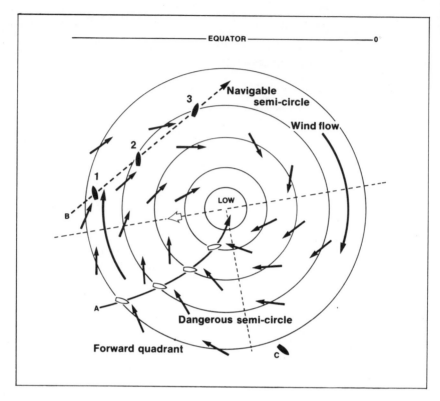

Fig. 126 *The dangerous and navigable semi-circles, Southern Hemisphere*

would have to pay off to port with the successive wind shifts on the storm's approach. If this were not done a boat could literally sail itself into the path of the storm if not into the centre itself. Boat C on the fringes of the storm might only have received a minor buffeting and seems safe because the centre has moved past it to the west. However, C could find itself directly ahead of the eye if the storm recurved. For these reasons, the area on the inside of the curve in both hemispheres is called the dangerous semi-circle.

In the semi-circle closest to the equator in both hemispheres, i.e., on the outside of the curve, the effect of the winds ahead of the storm is to drift a boat such as B out of the direct path of the approaching centre. In addition, the centre will move away from the equator and thus the boat if there is any recurvature. So the left semi-circle in the Northern Hemisphere and the right semi-circle in the Southern Hemisphere are called the *navigable semi-circles*. This does not mean that the winds are any the less strong, but at least a boat has a sporting chance of avoiding the worst of the storm.

150

Warning signs

The use of weather satellites and radar-equipped aircraft has greatly increased the weather forecasters' ability to detect and track the progress of tropical storms. This information is broadcast to the public on radio and television and to the boat owner by coast radio stations. In fact gale and cyclone warnings are usually transmitted as soon as they are received. Without this type of information there is no guaranteed method of predicting the approach of a tropical cyclone but to anyone in an area subject to these storms, especially in the season, the following are good indications that one might be approaching.

Local weather may be unusually good on the day before the storm, with a higher than normal barometer reading and almost cloudless skies. For all the apparent indications of a continuing fine spell, it *feels* wrong. This is hardly a scientific appraisal, I know, but the weather can become oppressively humid. Although any prevailing wind will be causing a slight sea, there may be a long low swell coming from a different direction. If suspicions are aroused, the barometer should be read every two or three hours. There is always a small variation above and below the mean atmospheric pressure each day and this can be found in a climatic atlas or the *Sailing Directions* for the particular area and the particular time of year.

A fall of 3 millibars below normal pressure is a bad sign and a fall of 5 or more millibars below normal means that a tropical storm is almost certainly lurking nearby. Three millibars does not sound very much in itself, but the cyclone season is in the summer months and, taken together with the time of year, the place and the usually small diurnal variation in pressure, it is most significant.

As time passes, leading to the day of the storm, the swell may build up with a frequency of two to five crests each minute, compared with the more usual ten to fifteen crests each minute. High cirrus clouds start to appear from the direction of the storm centre, and by this stage a moderate wind will be blowing. Any appreciable and sudden changes in wind strength or direction give further warning of the approach of a tropical cyclone. Several hours after the first high clouds appear, the cloud bases will progressively lower, bringing substantially increasing winds with frequent rain and the barometer will continue to fall.

This description of events sounds very much like those experienced in the approach of warm and cold front depression. However, the sequence is over a very much shorter period of time with a faster-falling barometer and a quicker onset of gale force winds and weather.

Avoiding a tropical cyclone

Once it is clear that a boat at sea is in the vicinity of a tropical storm, it is almost vital to find the direction of the centre if any avoiding action is to be taken. As with a middle latitude depression, this can be done by facing into the wind. The centre of low pressure then lies between 110° and 115° on the right hand in the Northern Hemisphere or the left hand in the Southern Hemisphere. The natural inclination might be to crack on all sail and try to get the hell out of there, but the recommended action is to heave-to for a while until the path of the centre is found by watching the wind shifts carefully and the movement of the barometer. With a falling pressure, the centre is getting closer, and with a rising pressure it is moving away. If the direction of the centre remains constant with a falling barometer, the vessel is in the direct path of the eye. There is little point in trying to outrun the storm in this case because tropical cyclones move somewhat faster than do most yachts. In other cases the change in the bearing of the centre over, say, a six-hour period will indicate the direction of the storm's movement. This information, combined with the direction of the wind shifts, should enable the navigator to decide in which part of which semi-circle the boat lies.

To illustrate the point, look at boat B in Fig. 126. With the boat at position 1, the centre would lie almost due E and the wind would be from the SSW. As the storm moved to the west, the boat would get closer to the centre. At position 2, the bearing of the centre would have changed to almost SE. The wind would have backed to SW and increased, and the barometer would be falling. These facts should tell the navigator that he is ahead of the storm in the navigable semi-circle.

I have been through several typhoons in a big ship, a couple of West Indian hurricanes and the odd cyclone, but to my everlasting relief, I have not been caught in a tropical revolving storm in a yacht. I suspect that for any yachtsman caught in one, the most pressing consideration will be that of simple survival. Far from being able to choose suitable courses, the conditions may call for bare pole sailing with a long warp or sea anchor streamed and the yachtsman's uppermost thought being to get out of the mess alive. Nevertheless, for want of any more authoritative advice on what to do, the rules given to the old sailing ship captains seem to be as good a starting point as any.

When a boat with plenty of sea room is in the path of the storm and ahead of the centre, the suggested action is to make a dash for the navigable semi-circle with the wind well on the starboard quarter in the Northern Hemisphere or on the port quarter in the Southern Hemisphere. However, the compass course first set should be maintained until the boat is well clear, despite the subsequent wind shifts. The same course of action should be taken if the boat is already in the navigable semi-circle and ahead of the storm centre.

The most critical position is if the boat is in the forward quadrant of the dangerous semi-circle. As already discussed, a sailing vessel will continually be beaten by the wind and sea towards the path of the storm and may end up in the centre without being able to avoid it. The action here is to haul by the wind on the starboard tack in north latitudes and the port tack in south latitudes. Then keep coming up as the wind draws aft and carry sail as long as possible.

Heaving-to

The choice of tack when forced to heave-to can be critical. For example, if the boat is on a given tack and the wind shifts across the bow, the boat will be slammed over onto the opposite tack. As we are talking of winds ranging from 70 to 90 knots or higher, this type of manoeuvre can result in sails being blown out, dismasting or even taking a 360° roll, assuming the boat comes up at all. If on the other hand the wind shifts aft towards the stern, the boat can head up towards the wind. A general rule for sailing vessels is always to heave-to on whatever tack will mean that the wind shifts draw aft.

In the right semi-circle in both hemispheres as the storm centre overtakes and passes, the wind will constantly veer to the right. The rate at which the wind veers will increase as the centre approaches. Following the general rule, then, a vessel should heave-to on the starboard tack.

In the left semi-circle the wind will continually back to the left so the vessel should heave-to on the port tack. All these rules for taking evasive action when caught in a tropical revolving storm are summarised in Fig. 127.

Position	*Action if under sail*	*Hove-to*
Southern Hemisphere		
Left or dangerous semi-circle	Keep close-hauled on the port tack, make as much ground as possible.	Port tack
Right or navigable semi-circle	Bring the wind on the port quarter. Note the course and hold it.	Starboard tack
Ahead of the centre in the path of the storm	Bring the wind 20° on the port quarter (200° REL). Note the course and hold it, making a run for the navigable semi-circle.	As above, depending on which semi-circle the craft is in at the time.
Behind the centre	Steer the best riding course to open out the distance from the centre, remembering that the cyclone may recurve to the south and east.	

Fig. 127 *Avoiding a tropical cyclone. If the recommended action will take the boat towards land or shoals, the only alternative is to heave-to on the appropriate tack.*

153

Chapter Ten
Navigating in Fog

A collision at sea can spoil your whole day.
Thucydides, Greek naval historian, 420 BC

In clear weather the navigator may not know his exact position, but with nearby vessels in sight and a coastline clearly visible there is a certain feeling of reassurance. However, when a good, hard horizon softens and then disappears, followed first by the more distant vessels and then by the land and closest craft as a silent wall of sea mist or fog envelopes the area, this feeling of well-being vanishes. If readers think that I am laying it on a bit thick — no pun intended — they have not had the responsibility for the safety of a boat in fog. Many readers may have leapfrogged from navigation mark to navigation mark in harbour or river mist, which can have its moments of excitement, but to be under way off a busy coastline in zero visibility is a different matter. Prevention being better than cure, it is unwise to go to sea in fog or if the weather man is forecasting fog.

If it is necessary to go out, or if you are already at sea when visibility deteriorates, the navigator whose boat is fitted with radio aids such as a D/F set, radar or Decca navigator in those areas with Decca coverage, should be able to fix your position. Without these aids you must rely on two sources of information — your depth finder and your ears.

The hard facts must be accepted that the boat is in a dangerous situation where the possibilities of collision and grounding may be very real. The most important consideration becomes the safety of those on board and this may depend on certain precautions being taken. Life jackets should be donned and a lookout should be placed right forward in the bows. If the boat is under power, this lookout, who should be as far away as possible from engine noise, will double as the crew member primarily responsible for listening for the fog signals of other vessels. This duty should be rotated every half hour because efficiency falls off rapidly after this period of time. The depth finder should be put into action. Unnecessary lighting should be turned off because it reduces visibility even further by reflecting back off the fog. If the boat is under

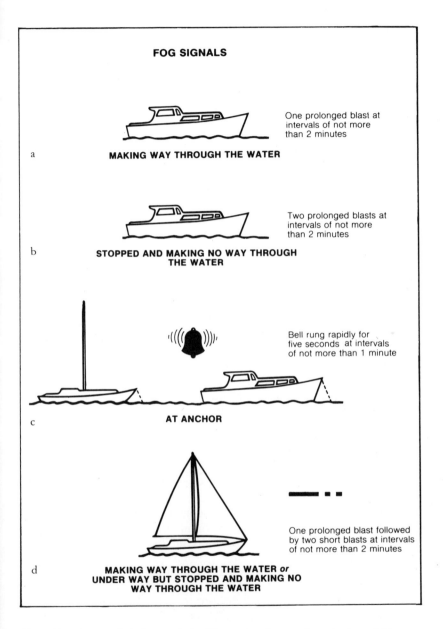

Fig. 128a, b, c and d *Fog signals. These signals may be substituted by some other efficient sound signal at intervals of not more than 2 minutes for vessels of less than 12 m in length. (Adapted from* Safety in Small Craft, *NZ Govt. Printer in conjunction with the Ministry of Transport*

sail, the engine should be run up and tested ready for immediate use.

Speed must be reduced in accordance with the regulations for the prevention of collision at sea, and the correct fog signal started. These fog signals are shown in Fig. 128. Remember that, if the boat is under sail and the engine is used at a later stage, the fog signal must be changed from that for a yacht to the signal for a power boat of equivalent length, even if the sails are left hoisted.

Vessels less than 12 metres in length may substitute some other efficient sound signal at intervals of not more than 2 minutes. Using a hand held whistle or banging a pot with a hammer are possibilities.

The other important rule to do with restricted visibility states that 'Except where it has been determined that a risk of collision does not exist, every vessel that hears apparently forward of her beam the fog signal of another vessel, or which cannot avoid a close quarters situation with another vessel forward of her beam, shall reduce speed to the minimum at which she can be kept on her course. She shall if necessary take all her way off and in any event navigate with extreme caution until danger of collision is over.'

Briefly, this means that a boat fitted with radar may be able to tell that there is no danger of collision with other vessels ahead. All other boats must slow so that they barely have steerage way and must stop if necessary until the situation has been sorted out. If this means that two or more vessels have to stay stopped in thick fog for a long period because they are unsure of each other's positions, only to find when the fog thins that they were perfectly safe because they were all heading away from each other, then so be it. The regulations are designed to stop ships colliding in reduced visibility. They give no guarantee that vessels will travel from A to B in the shortest possible time.

Position

As to position finding in fog, the navigator may have to rely on dead reckoning or using an estimated position. One factor can act to the navigator's advantage; in thick weather, when there is little or no wind, tidal streams or currents should be the same as or very close to their predicted directions and speeds. Estimated positions based on this information should therefore be more reliable than those calculated in rough weather.

If the boat is in enclosed waters or in a channel, the visiblity can be gauged by reading the log to find the distance travelled between the time of passing a buoy and the time it disappears in the fog. This information can be used to estimate the expected time of sighting succeeding buoys or marks.

When sailing off the coast and if shore marks are in sight prior to the visibility closing in, it is important to start the period of blind navigation from as accurate and up-to-date a position as possible. The

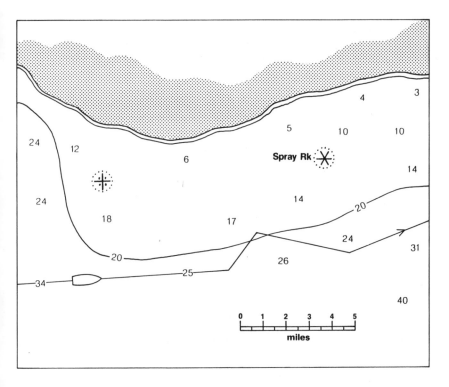

Fig. 129 *Use of depth contour to parallel coastline*

latest fix on the chart should be only minutes old when the fixing marks merge into the mist. After that, it may be possible to run a safe course roughly parallel to the coast, by using a depth contour as a clearing line. For example, in Fig. 129 the 20-metre line is about four miles offshore. The depth falls away sharply to over 30 metres. There are no dangers more than 3 miles from the coast. If the boat stays in depths of 20 metres or more there is no danger of grounding. If it was on a long coastal passage, it would be wise to turn back into the 20-metre line every so often to ensure that the craft was not being slowly set out to sea.

Conversely, the navigator who wishes to close the coast from seaward can attempt to run a line of soundings, as explained on page 100. Other options dependent on the circumstances include hauling back out to sea or anchoring. If the visibility is a few hundred metres the navigator may be prepared to stand well in to the coast, either to anchor or to continue cautiously in shallow water. But if there are off-lying dangers further along the intended track, there should be no half measures – the navigator should either go well inside them, hugging the shoreline, or stay out in deep water.

Shore fog signals

In harbour some wharves or jetties and navigation marks are fitted with fog signals, as are certain coastal lights and offshore buoys. The various instruments used and the abbreviations found on charts are: diaphone (Dia), siren, reed, gun, explosive (Explos), bell, gong or whistle (Whis). Three older terms — electric fog horn, nautophone (Nauto) and tyfon — will in future be described under the general heading 'horn', but will continue to be found on charts that have not been converted to metric units. The diaphone, siren and reed are all compressed air instruments. Bells may be operated mechanically or by the action of the waves; in which case they are unlikely to work in calm seas.

On approaching a coast, the navigator is usually advised to make for one of the lights fitted with a fog signal, the theory being that hearing its sound will help him establish his position. The rider is also added that there should be a depth contour that can be used as a limiting line, i.e., if the signal has not been heard by the time the craft is in a given depth, the approach should be broken off while still in safe water. The reason for this is that sound waves can be distorted in mist or fog and the signals are heard at varying distances. Signals that are clearly audible at, say, a mile or so from a light may be inaudible at half a mile. The distortion also means that the apparent direction of the signal's source is markedly different to the true direction of the light. Other qualifications are that the boat may have to be stopped from time to time because engine noise may drown out a weak signal, or in larger boats that it may be heard by someone up the mast but not by those on deck.

For those people who have no option, but must return to harbour, the earlier suggestion that they make for a coastal lighthouse is no doubt sound advice. However, on a busy coast the odds are that all the other vessels, large and small, are also blindly homing in on the fog signal. The area could become as congested as a Friday night traffic snarl. Due to the greatly increased possibility of collision or near collision, and given any flexibility in my time of arrival, I would take my chances somewhere else.

Distance off by echo

If the boat is in the vicinity of high cliffs or a bluff headland, the navigator may be warned of too close an approach by having his fog signals echoed back from the cliffs. The approximate distance can be found in such circumstances in that nine-tenths of the total time in seconds equals the distance in tenths of a mile: e.g., a boat that hears the echo after 10 seconds is nine-tenths or 0.9 of a mile from the cliff. If the echo returns after three and a half seconds, the distance is $(3.5 \times 0.9) \div 10$, or 0.3 miles.

The echo technique should be used only to give warning of too close an approach to the coast, not to prove that the boat is a safe distance off. Even so, an adaptation can be used if visibility decreases sharply as a boat is passing between steep headlands on its way in or out of harbour. If the boat is midway between the cliffs, the echo from each side should be heard at the same time. As long as the channel is also in the centre of the gap between the cliffs, the boat can be kept in mid-channel by turning away from the echo that returns first until the two are again heard together. Warning: If the channel is closer to one cliff than the other do not use this technique.

Checklist in fog

Before discussing the use of radar in thick weather and at other times, the checklist given below could be a useful reference to all boat owners. These precautions should be put into effect before entering fog.

1. Obtain fix by visual means if possible.
2. Confirm that the helmsman knows the compass course, and instruct him to maintain as accurate a heading as possible for dead reckoning purposes.
3. Start depth finder.
4. Reduce to moderate speed.
5. If under sail, prepare engine for immediate use.
6. Switch on normal navigation lights, day or night, but reduce all other lighting to a minimum.
7. Place a lookout in the bows.
8. Ensure that the radar reflector is hoisted if one is carried.
9. Instruct all crew members to don life jackets and to keep absolute silence on deck.
10. In shoal waters, have an anchor ready for letting go.
11. Note other vessels in the vicinity so that their fog signals do not catch you by surprise.
12. Ensure that flares, life raft/dinghy and other emergency equipment is ready for immediate use.
13. On entering the fog, start the prescribed fog signal.
14. The navigator must continually assess safe courses and maintain an accurate EP, anchoring if the situation warrants it.

Radar fixing

Radar is fitted in more and more small boats these days and it is a valuable aid to navigation in restricted visibility or at night. It is outside the scope of this book to explain the principles involved or the operation of the radar displays; I intend rather to explain the use of radar information in position finding.

Most small-boat radars have radar relative displays such as that shown in Fig. 130a, where the 0° to 360° bearing ring is used to read off relative bearings. The vertical line from the centre of the display is the boat's heading marker, and always reads 0°, regardless of the boat's actual course. So the nearest point of land shown in Fig. 130a is on the boat's starboard bow, at about 030° REL. If the craft altered course to head for the land, the radar picture would rotate counter-clockwise and then steady, with the land echo straddling the heading marker, i.e., dead ahead at 0° REL.

Radar is not infallible. It is subject to atmospheric conditions, like any other radio wave, and must be used with a certain amount of caution. Large steel ships and bold cliffy coastlines give excellent echoes; wooden or GRP boats tend to absorb the radar beams and are poor targets. The owners of such craft would be wise to have a radar reflector fitted to greatly enhance their chances of being detected by larger vessels. Low, sandy coastlines may not show up on radar displays except at very short distances.

Mountain tops or hills may be seen above the horizon before the coast and shoreline come into view and they are also visible on radar. High land, which may be well inshore, appears on the display first. When the boat closes the coast, the picture slowly fills in as the low-lying land or shoreline is detected. The danger here is that the navigator may believe that he is two or three miles from the shore when he is actually that distance from some higher ground inland. He would thus be closer to the shore with its possible dangers than the radar range has indicated.

Most large navigational buoys have radar reflectors fitted to ensure that the marks show up clearly on the radar screen. On older charts any buoys so fitted were identified by having a symbol over the top that looked like a spiky crown. These days it is assumed that all channel marking buoys, certainly in the IALA system, have radar reflectors, and the symbol is being phased out.

Mind you, another small boat gives much the same echo as a buoy on the radar screen. To overcome this problem, certain buoys are self-identifying on radar. One type is the Racon which is marked on a chart with a magenta ring around it. The buoy is fitted with a radar transmitter triggered by the pulse from a ship's radar. The returning echo shows up as a bar on the screen and the end nearest the vessel is the Racon's position. A second type, the Ramark, is not triggered by ship's radar but transmits continuously. The echo appears as a broken line.

Although most radars give both the bearing and distance of detected objects, the distance reading is the more accurate because of the nature of the radar beam. So, when finding position with radar, the most reliable results are gained by using range arc fixes described on page 116. It is safest to use ranges of prominent headlands or small steep-cliffed islands for the reasons given earlier. Newer charts are being printed with radar prominent areas clearly shaded on the coastlines. These are areas that show up distinctly on radar screens. For example, Fig. 130b shows part of a chart with radar prominent areas shaded in. The navigator has used the radar ranges of Bluff Point (2 miles), the Finger (3.5 miles), and the

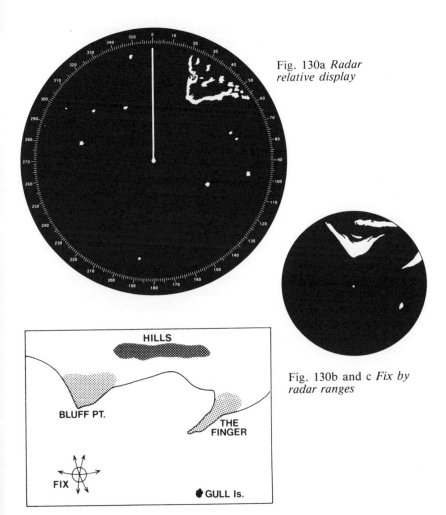

Fig. 130a *Radar relative display*

Fig. 130b and c *Fix by radar ranges*

HILLS

BLUFF PT.

THE FINGER

FIX

● GULL Is.

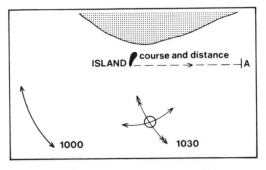

ISLAND ⬩ course and distance

A

1000

1030

Fig. 131 *Running fix using two range arcs*

closest edge of Gull Island (3.6 miles) to plot the range arc fix shown. Fig. 130c shows the radar picture.

There may be only one identifiable point or island on the radar during a given period. A running fix can be used here by transferring the first range arc up to the time of the second. Sure, they are both curves, but the problem is overcome by using the procedure illustrated in Fig. 131. The first step is to take the radar range, noting the time and log reading. Plot the arc on the chart. Some time later, read off a second range and plot it, also noting the time and log reading. To transfer the first arc, lay off the boat's course and distance travelled by log from the *island or prominent point used* when taking the ranges. This gives point A in the diagram. Using this point as the centre, and setting the initial range on the dividers, lay off an arc. The point at which this cuts the second is the running fix. In other words, the problem of moving a curve is solved by moving the centre of the circle and redrawing the curve.

Conversely, a range arc from one object can be transferred in the same manner to give a fix by crossing it with the range arc from a different object taken at a later time, as explained on page 88.

A radar picture needs a certain amount of interpretation and the navigator will not gain this skill by leaving the thing switched off except very occasionally when the boat is in fog or the visibility deteriorates. As with any unfamiliar technique, the use of radar fixing needs to be practised if the navigator is to gain confidence in it. This practice should take place in good weather, when the boat can be fixed by visual means and radar fixes taken at the same time compared with these positions.

Radar clearing range

As with the clearing bearing in visual navigation, it is not always necessary to fix the boat's position when using radar to ensure that it is in safe water. A radar clearing range does the same job as the clearing bearing, or, more accurately, the same job as the danger angle. The technique is to measure the distance between the danger and the nearest radar prominent land on the chart. Then choose a safety margin of, say, a half to one mile, and add this to the distance. As long as the land echo on the radar screen is outside this total distance, the boat is safe. The navigator can check this by glancing at the radar from time to time. No measurement or plotting is needed, nor need the boat remain on a steady course.

An example is given in Fig. 132. Horn Rock is 4.5 miles from Little Barrier and is a danger at night or in fog. The island has steep cliffs that give good radar echoes. Any boat working to the south-east of the island would be safe as long as it did not approach within 5 miles; conversely, it would also be in clear water if it remained 4 miles or closer to Little Barrier. Fig. 132b shows the radar scope and the circle indicates a range of 5 miles. The island is clearly at a greater range. However, in Fig 132c the boat has closed with the land which is exactly 5 miles away. The boat may be within half a mile of Horn Rock and the navigator would regain safe water by turning away from the land and opening out the distance.

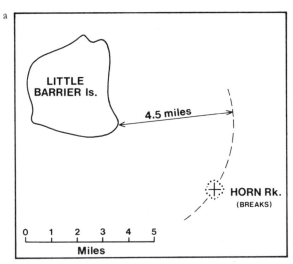

Fig. 132a, b and c
*Using a 5-mile radar
clearing range to
avoid Horn Rock*

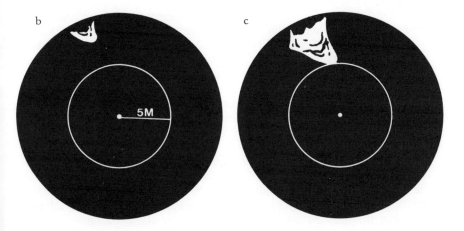

Appendix 1
Radio Aids

There are a number of radio aids to navigation but all of them need certain specialised receivers, or gridded charts may have to be used before a fix can be plotted. The basic radio aid consists of an omnidirectional transmitter sited onshore called a radio beacon, and a receiver on board which is linked to an aerial that can be used to sense the direction or bearing of the beacon from the boat. The process of finding direction in this way is called radio direction finding, or RDF. If the receiving aerial can have a compass incorporated or be compared in some manner with the steering compass, a true bearing can be worked out and plotted on a chart in the same way as is the visual bearing of a navigation mark. Plotting the bearings of two or more radio beacons gives a fix.

These beacons have been set up at strategic points along the coast, primarily for the use of RDF-fitted vessels in finding position during periods of fog or low visibility, and at other times when a vessel is too far off the coast to see visual fixing marks. Many give a continuous 24-hour service, some operate solely at night and others are only switched on during periods of fog or restricted visibility.

Most marine radio beacons operate in the frequency range 285 kHz to 320 kHz, each station being identified by a characteristic call sign of one or more letters of the alphabet. World-wide details of marine beacons can be found in volume II of the *Admiralty List of Radio Signals*. National details are contained in publications such as *Reed's Almanac* (United Kingdom) and the *NZ Nautical Almanac*. Radio beacons can be identified on charts by a magenta (purple) circle with the abbreviation RC alongside. Those circles marked Aero RC are intended for aircraft use, but they can be used by surface craft as discussed later.

In certain areas, groups of between two and six beacons operate on the same frequency and transmit one at a time in succession. This assists the navigator to get a fix because no tuning is needed between stations when bearings are being taken.

Aerials
Two types of direction sensing aerials are used with RDF equipment.

164

Both types can be rotated through 360° and the signal, heard either through earphones or indicated on a meter, will vary from a maximum to a minimum strength. The older vertical loop aerial gives maximum volume when edge-on to the transmitting station and minimum signal strength when facing directly towards the radio beacon. The more recent horizontal ferrite rod aerial is the reverse of this, giving a maximum signal when broadside-on and a minimum signal when pointing directly towards a station.

If the aerial is rotated, the rate of change of signal strength is greatest as it falls to a minimum. The aerial and receiver are coupled in such a way that direction is determined with the signal at minimum strength. In fact, when using either type of aerial the signal can be lost altogether, and this is called the *null* point. When aerials are turned through a full circle, there may be two null points approximately 180° apart. This leads to a bearing ambiguity and the approximate bearing of a station must first be found from the boat's DR or EP on the chart.

Bearings

Aerials are either portable or attached to the boat's superstructure, with a 360° scale fitted beneath. A pointer directly attached to the aerial moves around the scale as the latter is rotated and direction is read off against the pointer. The scale is mounted with the zero forward, and the 0°–180° line either along or parallel to the fore and aft line of the boat.

When the minimum signal or null point is reached, the bearing of the beacon *relative* to the bow of the craft may be found.

However, to turn this relative bearing into an accurate true bearing, it is essential to know the boat's heading at the moment the bearing is read off. The heading at that time may differ by several degrees from the course being steered.

Fig. 133 *Coast refraction*

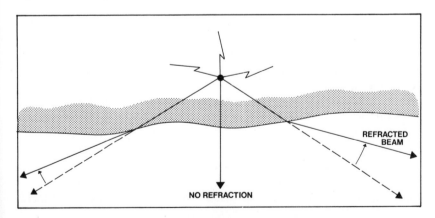

Another method is to use a rotatable scale with a lubber line set up in the boat's fore and aft line. When the null point is found, this scale is rotated until the heading by steering compass is opposite the lubber line and the scale locked in position. This means that the *compass bearing* of the radio beacon may be read directly from the scale.

Probably the most useful instrument for the small craft navigator is the hand-held ferrite rod type, fitted with a compass. This is a completely portable RDF set. The aerial and compass are rotated together and the compass bearing of the station is read directly when the null point is found.

Example: The relative bearing of a radio beacon, taken in a boat on course 080°C, is found to be 120°REL. Variation is 8°E and deviation on course 080°C is 2°W. To find the true bearing of the beacon, the boat's course is first converted to true, and then the relative bearing is added.

Compass course	080°C
Deviation	− 2°W
Magnetic course	078°M
Variation	+ 8°E
True course	086°T
Relative bearing	+120°REL
True bearing	206°T

Limitations

Some readers will know that certain areas around the coasts of their own countries are notorious for giving unreliable results when using RDF. This sort of local knowledge cannot be covered here, but there are some general effects which can induce errors in RDF bearings, and the reader should be aware of these limitations.

Night distortion

During the period from about one hour before sunset to one hour after sunrise, skywave signals received via the ionosphere from stations more than 25 miles from the vessel can distort the more direct ground wave transmissions, leading to inaccurate bearings. Inside 25 miles this error is unlikely to arise. The effect is worst around sunrise and sunset and RDF sets should not be used at these times. Any positions obtained during the night using RDF which differ markedly from a good EP should be regarded with extreme suspicion.

Coast refraction

It is advisable to consult the chart to find the path of the transmissions from any given RDF station. If high land intervenes or if the radio wave will cross the coastline at a fine angle or even parallel to the coast, errors are likely. In the last two cases the radio wave will be bent, or refracted, back towards the coast as shown in Fig. 133. There is no refraction when waves cross the coast at right angles.

Quadrantal error

This error is due to radio waves being reflected off a vessel's mast, rigging or superstructure into the receiving aerial. These reflected waves distort the direct beam from the radio beacon. The aerial interprets this combined beam as coming from a slightly different direction than that in which the beacon actually lies, giving an incorrect bearing. The effect is virtually nil when the station is ahead, astern or on the beam, but is at a maximum when it is 45° either side of the bow or stern.

Calibration

If the RDF aerial is mounted permanently, quadrantal error can be found by comparing the visual bearings of a radio beacon and those obtained at the same time with the RDF set.

The craft should be stationed from 3 to 5 miles from the beacon, slowly turning through a full circle and steadying at every 20° heading change. Two people will probably be needed, one to take the visual bearings with an HBC while the other operates the RDF set. When the craft is steady, the RDF bearing is found and at the same time the compass bearing of the station is found and the boat's heading by steering compass is noted. The last two findings are converted to magnetic directions, and comparison of the two gives the relative bearing of the radio beacon. This is compared with the relative bearing given by the RDF set and any difference is due to quadrantal error, e.g.:

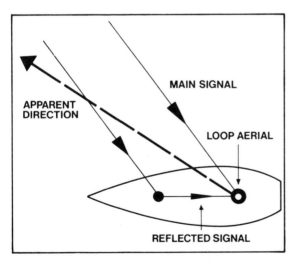

Fig. 134 *Quadrantal error*

MAIN SIGNAL

APPARENT
DIRECTION

LOOP AERIAL

REFLECTED SIGNAL

167

Heading by steering compass	130°C
Deviation (say)	−2°W
Magnetic heading	128°M
Magnetic bearing of radio beacon (HBC)	168°M
Relative bearing	(168°M − 128°M)
	40°REL
RDF relative bearing (say)	44°REL
Error	4° High (−)

A quadrantal error card, similar to a compass deviation card, can be drawn up. Although a similar table of errors may be made for a combined portable RDF set and compass, the navigator should realise that it is correct only for the exact spot on board the boat used when making up the error card. If RDF bearings are subsequently obtained when standing at some other place, the quadrantal errors could be different to those noted on the card.

Aeronautical radio beacons
Certain radio beacons designed primarily for aircraft use are situated near the coast and may be useful for surface craft. Other aero beacons situated well inland may often be heard at sea, but the radio wave may be distorted by coastal refraction and other land effects, especially if there are intervening high hills.

Tidal Calculations

The height of tide at intermediate times between high and low water can be found using the Rule of Twelfths (see page 28) but more accurate results can be obtained by using the special methods given in national tide tables. Unlike most other procedures in coastal navigation, the method of working out heights of tide at any given time differs slightly from country to country. What follows is an explanation of those used in New Zealand.

TIDE TABLES

The Range Table shown in Fig. 135 is taken from the *New Zealand Tide Tables*. The table contains four headings, i.e., duration of rise or fall, range in metres, interval from the nearest high (or low) water and a correction to the height of high (or low) water. If any three of these are known, the fourth can be found from the table.

The first step in finding the height of tide at a given time is to take the data for the high and low water either side of this time from the tables. Then find the duration and range of this tide and the interval between the required time and the nearer of the times of high or low water. The range table is entered by finding the duration in the left hand column and the interval along the line immediately to the right in the main part of the table. By dropping down this column to the bottom part of the table and opposite the range, the correction to the height of the nearest high or low water is found. This correction is added to the height of low water or subtracted from the height of high water, depending on which is nearest to the given time.

For example, to find the height of tide at 0518 at Auckland when the data from the tables are:

0315	0.4
1005	3.4
1554	0.3
2232	3.5

0518 is between the time of LW at 0315 and the HW at 1005. It is closest to the time of LW.

Predicted time of HW	1005
Predicted time of LW	0315
Duration	0650
Height of HW	3.4
Height of LW	0.4
Range	3.0
Required time	0518
Time of nearest tide (LW)	0315
Interval from LW	0203

Using these three values, the correction from the range table is 0.6 m. As it is based on LW and the tide is rising, the correction is added to the LW height.

Predicted height of LW at 0315	0.4
Correction to height of LW	0.6
Predicted height at 0518	1.0

Secondary ports

Tidal information for secondary ports is given immediately following the predictions for the standard ports in the *New Zealand Tide Tables*. The predictions for each place are shown as time differences to be added to or subtracted from the times of high and low water at a particular standard port. The heights of tides at spring and neap are tabulated against the spring and neap heights at the same standard port. At other times the heights of high and low water at the secondary port fall between the values listed.

Look at Fig. 136, which is an extract from the *NZTT*. The tides at Tryphena are 8 minutes earlier than those at the standard port, Auckland. On the other hand, the HW at Nagle Cove is 24 minutes earlier than at Auckland and the LW only 11 minutes earlier, e.g., to find the times of the tides at Nagle Cove based on the following data for Auckland:

0156	3.2
0807	0.6
1414	3.0
2036	0.6

	HW	HW	LW	LW
Predicted times at Auckland	0156	1414	0807	2036
Time differences at Nagle Cove	−0024	−0024	−0011	−0011
Predicted times at Nagle Cove	0132	1350	0756	2025

When NZDT is in force between the last Sunday in October and the first Sunday in March, 1 hour must be added to the predicted times.

To find the heights of HW and LW the Conversion Data given on the right hand side of the table is used. This consists of a high and low water multiplier (H.Mult. & L.Mult.) and a high and low water constant (H.Con. & L.Con.) The heights of the tides at the standard port are multiplied by the requisite multiplier, and then the particular constants are added to or subtracted from the result to give the heights of the tides at the secondary port.

Continuing with the example:

	HW	HW	LW	LW
Predicted heights at Auckland	3.2	3.0	0.6	0.6
H.Mult/L.Mult	×0.67	0.67	0.50	0.50
=	2.14	2.01	0.3	0.3
H.Con/L.Con	+0.23	0.23	0.1	0.1
Predicted heights at Nagle Cove	2.37	2.24	0.4	0.4

Tides at Nagle Cove:
0132	2.4
0756	0.4
1350	2.2
2025	0.4

Heights of tide in between high and low water can be worked out using the Range Table, in exactly the same way as for Standard Ports.

RANGE TABLE

*FOR FINDING THE HEIGHT OF THE TIDE AT TIMES BETWEEN
HIGH AND LOW WATER*

INTERVAL FROM NEAREST LOW WATER (HIGH WATER)

Duration of rise or fall																				
0400	0006	0012	0018	0024	0030	0036	0042	0048	0054	0100	0106	0112	0118	0124	0130	0136	0142	0148	0154	0200
10	0006	0013	0019	0025	0031	0038	0044	0050	0056	0103	0109	0115	0121	0128	0134	0140	0146	0153	0159	0205
20	0007	0013	0020	0026	0033	0039	0046	0052	0059	0105	0112	0118	0125	0131	0138	0144	0151	0157	0204	0210
30	0007	0014	0020	0027	0034	0041	0047	0054	0101	0108	0114	0121	0128	0135	0141	0148	0155	0202	0208	0215
40	0007	0014	0021	0028	0035	0042	0049	0056	0103	0110	0117	0124	0131	0138	0145	0152	0159	0206	0213	0220
0450	0007	0015	0022	0029	0036	0044	0051	0058	0105	0113	0120	0127	0134	0142	0149	0156	0203	0211	0218	0225
0500	0008	0015	0023	0030	0038	0045	0053	0100	0108	0115	0123	0130	0138	0145	0153	0200	0208	0215	0223	0230
10	0008	0016	0023	0031	0039	0047	0054	0102	0110	0118	0125	0133	0141	0149	0156	0204	0212	0220	0227	0235
20	0008	0016	0024	0032	0040	0048	0056	0104	0112	0120	0128	0136	0144	0152	0200	0208	0216	0224	0232	0240
30	0008	0017	0025	0033	0041	0050	0058	0106	0114	0123	0131	0139	0147	0156	0204	0212	0220	0229	0237	0245
40	0009	0017	0026	0034	0043	0051	0100	0108	0117	0125	0134	0142	0151	0159	0208	0216	0225	0233	0242	0250
0550	0009	0018	0026	0035	0044	0053	0101	0110	0119	0128	0136	0145	0154	0203	0211	0220	0226	0238	0246	0255
0600	0009	0018	0027	0036	0045	0054	0103	0112	0121	0130	0139	0148	0157	0206	0215	0224	0233	0242	0251	0300
10	0009	0019	0028	0037	0046	0056	0105	0114	0123	0133	0142	0151	0200	0210	0219	0228	0237	0247	0256	0305
20	0010	0019	0029	0038	0048	0057	0107	0116	0126	0135	0145	0154	0204	0213	0223	0232	0242	0251	0301	0310
30	0010	0020	0029	0039	0049	0059	0108	0118	0128	0138	0147	0157	0207	0217	0226	0236	0246	0256	0305	0315
40	0010	0020	0030	0040	0050	0100	0110	0120	0130	0140	0150	0200	0210	0220	0230	0240	0250	0300	0310	0320
0650	0010	0021	0031	0041	0051	0102	0112	0122	0132	0143	0153	0203	0213	0224	0234	0244	0254	0305	0315	0325
0700	0011	0021	0032	0042	0053	0103	0114	0124	0135	0145	0156	0206	0217	0227	0238	0248	0259	0309	0320	0330
10	0011	0022	0032	0043	0054	0105	0115	0126	0137	0148	0158	0209	0220	0231	0241	0252	0303	0314	0324	0335
20	0011	0022	0033	0044	0055	0106	0117	0128	0139	0150	0201	0212	0223	0234	0245	0256	0307	0318	0329	0340
30	0011	0023	0034	0045	0056	0108	0119	0130	0141	0153	0204	0215	0226	0238	0249	0300	0311	0323	0334	0345
40	0012	0023	0035	0046	0058	0109	0121	0132	0144	0155	0207	0218	0230	0241	0253	0304	0316	0327	0339	0350
0750	0012	0024	0035	0047	0059	0111	0122	0134	0146	0158	0209	0221	0233	0245	0256	0308	0320	0332	0343	0355
0800	0012	0024	0036	0048	0100	0112	0124	0136	0148	0200	0212	0224	0236	0248	0300	0312	0324	0336	0348	0400

The table below reproduces Fig. 135. The horizontal axis is the Range (M); each row is one correction column, giving the correction (in metres) to the height of low water (or high water) for the stated range.

Range M →	0.2	0.4	0.6	0.8	1.0	1.2	1.4	1.6	1.8	2.0	2.2	2.4	2.6	2.8	3.0	3.2	3.4	3.6	3.8	4.0	4.2	4.4	4.6	4.8	5.0
	0.1	0.2	0.3	0.4	0.5	0.6	0.7	0.8	0.9	1.0	1.1	1.2	1.3	1.4	1.5	1.6	1.7	1.8	1.9	2.0	2.1	2.2	2.3	2.4	2.5
	0.1	0.2	0.3	0.4	0.5	0.6	0.6	0.7	0.8	0.9	1.0	1.1	1.2	1.3	1.4	1.5	1.6	1.6	1.7	1.8	1.9	2.0	2.1	2.2	2.3
	0.1	0.2	0.3	0.3	0.4	0.5	0.6	0.7	0.8	0.8	0.9	1.0	1.1	1.2	1.3	1.4	1.4	1.5	1.6	1.7	1.8	1.9	1.9	2.0	2.1
	0.1	0.2	0.2	0.3	0.4	0.5	0.5	0.6	0.7	0.8	0.8	0.9	1.0	1.1	1.1	1.2	1.3	1.4	1.5	1.5	1.6	1.7	1.8	1.8	1.9
	0.1	0.1	0.2	0.2	0.3	0.4	0.5	0.6	0.6	0.7	0.8	0.8	0.9	0.9	1.0	1.1	1.2	1.2	1.3	1.4	1.5	1.5	1.6	1.7	1.7
	0.1	0.1	0.2	0.2	0.3	0.3	0.4	0.5	0.6	0.6	0.7	0.7	0.8	0.9	0.9	1.0	1.0	1.1	1.2	1.2	1.3	1.4	1.4	1.5	1.5
	0.0	0.1	0.2	0.2	0.3	0.3	0.4	0.4	0.5	0.5	0.6	0.7	0.7	0.8	0.8	0.9	0.9	1.0	1.0	1.1	1.1	1.2	1.3	1.3	1.4
	0.0	0.1	0.1	0.2	0.2	0.3	0.3	0.4	0.4	0.5	0.5	0.6	0.6	0.7	0.7	0.8	0.8	0.9	0.9	1.0	1.0	1.1	1.1	1.2	1.2
	0.0	0.1	0.1	0.1	0.2	0.2	0.3	0.3	0.4	0.4	0.5	0.5	0.6	0.6	0.7	0.7	0.8	0.8	0.9	0.9	1.0	1.0	1.1	1.1	1.2
	0.0	0.0	0.1	0.1	0.1	0.2	0.2	0.2	0.3	0.3	0.3	0.4	0.4	0.5	0.5	0.6	0.6	0.6	0.7	0.7	0.8	0.8	0.8	0.9	0.9
	0.0	0.0	0.0	0.1	0.1	0.1	0.1	0.2	0.2	0.2	0.3	0.3	0.3	0.3	0.4	0.4	0.4	0.5	0.5	0.5	0.6	0.6	0.6	0.7	0.7
	0.0	0.0	0.0	0.0	0.1	0.1	0.1	0.1	0.1	0.2	0.2	0.2	0.2	0.2	0.3	0.3	0.3	0.3	0.4	0.4	0.4	0.4	0.5	0.5	0.5
	0.0	0.0	0.0	0.0	0.0	0.0	0.1	0.1	0.1	0.1	0.1	0.1	0.1	0.2	0.2	0.2	0.2	0.2	0.3	0.3	0.3	0.3	0.3	0.4	0.4
	0.0	0.0	0.0	0.0	0.0	0.0	0.0	0.0	0.1	0.1	0.1	0.1	0.1	0.1	0.1	0.1	0.2	0.2	0.2	0.2	0.2	0.2	0.3	0.3	0.3
	0.0	0.0	0.0	0.0	0.0	0.0	0.0	0.0	0.0	0.0	0.0	0.0	0.0	0.0	0.0	0.0	0.0	0.0	0.0	0.0	0.0	0.0	0.0	0.0	0.0

Fig. 135 Range table for finding the height of the tide at times between high and low water

173

SECONDARY PORTS TABLE

Place	Lat. S.	Long. E	Time Differences M.H.W. (h. m.)	Time Differences M.L.W. (h. m.)	M.H. W.S.	M.H. W.N.	M.L. W.N.	M.L. W.S.	M.S.L.	H. Mult.	H. Con.	L. Mult.	L. Con.
AUCKLAND	36 51	174 46	-0022	+0032	3.1	2.8	0.8	0.4	1.8	1.00	0.00	1.00	0.00
†Mokohinau Island	35 54	175 07	-0022	-0001	2.3	2.1	0.6	0.3	1.3	0.67	0.23	0.75	0.00
Kawau Island													
Mansion House Bay	36 26	174 49	-0022	-0001	2.6	2.3	0.8	0.5	1.6	1.00	-0.50	0.75	0.20
West Side Hauraki Gulf													
†Matakana River	36 24	174 44	+0005	+0005	2.7	2.4	0.9	0.5	1.6	1.00	-0.40	1.00	0.10
†Mahurangi Harbour	36 29	174 43	+0002	+0012	◊	◊	◊	◊	◊	◊	◊	◊	◊
Tiritiri Matangi Is.	36 36	174 53	+0015	-0003	2.9	2.6	0.8	0.5	1.7	1.00	-0.20	0.75	0.20
Weiti River	36 39	174 44	-0003	+0007	2.8	2.5	0.9	0.6	1.7	1.00	-0.30	0.75	0.30
*Murrays Bay	36 44	174 45	-0025	-0003	2.9	2.6	0.8	0.5	1.7	1.00	-0.20	0.75	0.20
Waiheke Island													
Matiatia Bay	36 47	174 59	-0014	-0006	2.8	2.4	0.6	0.3	1.6	1.33	-1.33	0.75	-0.00
Man O'War Bay	36 47	175 09	-0021	-0003	3.0	2.6	0.7	0.3	1.6	1.33	-1.13	1.00	-0.10
Coromandel Peninsula													
Coromandel Harbour	36 47	175 25	-0016	-0006	2.8	2.5	0.8	0.5	1.7	1.00	-0.30	0.75	0.20
Rocky Point (Thames)	37 06	175 31	-0031	-0024	3.3	2.9	0.9	0.5	1.9	1.33	-0.83	1.00	0.10
Port Jackson	36 29	175 20	-0030	-0012	2.6	2.3	0.7	0.4	1.5	1.00	-0.50	0.75	0.10
Great Barrier Island													
Nagle Cove	36 09	175 21	-0024	-0011	2.3	2.1	0.5	0.3	1.3	0.67	0.23	0.50	0.10
Tryphena	36 19	175 29	-0008	-0008	2.26	2.02	0.72	0.48	1.37	1.00	-0.80	0.50	0.30
Kermadec Islands													
Raoul Island	29 15	178 05	-0033	-0025	1.4	1.2	0.4	0.2	0.8	0.67	-0.67	0.50	0.00

*Data Approximate.   ◊No Data.   †Time Indication Only.   ‡Time Differences Approximate.

Fig. 136 *Secondary ports: time differences and heights*

Glossary of Terms

abeam   In a direction at right angles to the longitudinal axis of a craft in the horizontal plane, i.e., 90° around from the bow on either side.

angle on the bow (AOB)   Horizontal angle between the bow of a boat and the direction of any external object measured from 0° to 180° to port or starboard (*see* relative direction).

Agonic line   A line joining points on the earth's surface where there is no magnetic variation.

awash   A rock, shoal or other danger is described on charts as awash when its highest point is exactly at the level of chart datum. In practical terms, the height of tide at any given moment is the depth of water over the danger.

back   The wind is said to back when it changes direction counter-clockwise.

broach to   To be carried inadvertently broadside on to the sea, when running before it.

beacon   A mark of solid construction erected on or in the vicinity of dangers, or onshore, as an aid to navigation.

bearing   The direction of one point from another.

buoys   Floats of standard colours and shapes moored as aids to navigation.

Buys-Ballot's Law   If an observer faces into the wind the centre of low pressure will lie between 100° to 110° on the left hand in the southern hemisphere, and on the right hand in the northern.

cardinal point   North, east, south, or west.

chart datum   The level below which depths are given on charts. Heights of tides are above chart datum. See LAT.

circle of error (of uncertainty)   An estimated error in position stated as a radial distance from a specific point.

claw off   To beat to windward away from a lee shore.

coasting   Navigating from headland to headland in sight of land, or often enough in sight of land to fix the position of the craft using land features.

cocked hat   The triangle resulting from the intersection of three position lines that do not meet at a point.

compass   An instrument used for indicating direction.

Cook Strait   Narrow body of water between north and south islands of New Zealand connecting Tasman Sea and Pacific Ocean.

course   The angle between the meridian through a craft and the fore and aft line, measured 0° to 360° clockwise from north. The intended direction of travel of a craft through the water in the horizontal plane (*see* heading).

course made good (CMG)   The mean course achieved.

cut (angle of)   The smaller angle between any two position lines.

datum   A horizontal plane to which heights, depths or levels are referred.

dead reckoning   Forecasting a boat's probable position based on course, speed and elapsed time.

dead reckoning position (DR)   The position resulting from dead reckoning.

Decca Navigator system   A low frequency system based on a phase comparison between a master and three slave stations.

departure   The east-west component of a rhumb line, measured in nautical miles.

deviation   Any angular deflection. In particular the angle between the direction of magnetic north and the direction of north given by a magnetic compass that has deviation.

dew point   The temperature to which air must be cooled to reach saturation.

diurnal   Having a period of, occurring in, or related to a day.

D.Lat.   The north-south component of a rhumb line, measured in nautical miles.

draught   Depth of water a boat draws or needs to float her.

drift   A small unwanted movement. In particular the effect on a boat of the motion of the water, usually from tidal stream.

drying height   Heights above chart datum of dangers that are periodically covered and exposed by the rise and fall of the tide. Chart abbreviations are Dr., dries (obsolete), or underlined figures shown near foreshores or over tidal mudflat areas.

estimated position   The DR position adjusted for the known or estimated drift due to current, tidal stream or leeway.

fetch   The straight distance a wave has travelled over the surface.

fix   A position found by two or more intersecting position lines.

fluxgate compass   A solid state electronic compass which uses the earth's magnetic field as the directional force.

Fohn wind   A local warm, dry wind that can occur on the lee side of a mountain range.

fore and aft line   The longitudinal axis of a boat. Generally the centre line between bow and stern.

foul ground   A limited area of the sea bed in comparatively shallow water, which is strewn with obstructions making it unsuitable for anchoring.

Fremantle Doctor   A strong sea breeze of up to 25 knots found in western Australia. It sets in just before midday in the summer months, bringing relief — hence the name 'doctor' — from the oppressively hot temperatures. Still known to some locals as the Fremantle Docker, because square-rigged vessels used it to enter port.

globigerina ooze   Ooze consisting of some mud, but mostly of the skeletons of various single-celled animals covered with a casing of carbonate of lime (foraminifera), common in the surface waters of the sea. Most of the foraminifera in the ooze are a spherical shelled organism called the globigerina.

gnomonic chart   A chart on the gnomonic projection. Great circles appear as straight lines, but rhumb line and parallels of latitude are curved.

great circle   A circle whose plane passes through the centre of the earth, dividing it into halves: the largest circle that can be drawn around the surface of the earth.

grid   A network of lines on a chart to which positions can be related.

ground position   The position on the earth vertically below a craft.

ground track   The actual path of a vessel over the ground.

gyro compass   A compass having one or more gyroscopes as the directive element, and indicates true north.

heading (ship's head)   The direction in which the bow is pointing at any given moment.

hectopascal (hPa)   A hectopascal is the unit of atmospheric pressure. Pressure, being a force, is strictly defined in terms of mass and acceleration. The unit of force is the newton ($kg.m/s^2$), and of pressure is the pascal (N/m^2).
   1 hPa $=$ 100 newtons/square metre $=$ 100 pascals or one millibar (mb).

heel   The short-term attitude in roll of a craft, caused by external forces.

homing   Navigation to a given point ahead of a craft by use of information coming from a point source, e.g. homing on a light, radio beacon, fog signal.

inversion   A layer in the atmosphere where over a short vertical distance the temperature either stabilises or increases with height, instead of decreasing.

isobar   Line on a weather map joining points of equal pressure.

isogonal   A line on a chart joining points that have the same magnetic variation.

Katabatic or valley wind   A local wind caused when cold, dense air flows down a slope when it cools, especially at night. Most significant with coastal snow-covered mountains where an off-shore wind can below from the seaward facing valleys, but also coming from the steep sides of fiords.

LAT — *Lowest Astronomical Tide*   The lowest tidal level which can be predicted to occur under average meteorological conditions and any combination of earth, sun and moon. Used as chart datum on metric charts.

latitude   Angular distance north or south of the equator, measured from 0° to 90°N or S at the centre of the earth.

leeway   Sideways movement of a boat through the water due to the effect of wind.

leg   The run made on a single tack, or any convenient length subdivision of a journey into a number of stages.

list   The long-term attitude in roll of a boat caused by internal forces.

local magnetic anomaly   A local effect superimposed on the earth's normal magnetic field, and noted on charts where it is known to exist. The practical effect is an alteration to the normal value of variation given on the particular chart.

log   An instrument that indicates boat speed and/or distance travelled through the water. It is also the document used as a boat's diary of events and includes a chronological record of the navigational progress of the craft.

longitude   Angular distance measured at the centre of the earth in the plane of the equator, between the Greenwich or prime meridian and the meridian through the place. Given in degrees, from 0° to 180°E or W.

loom   The diffused glow of a light seen when the light itself is below the horizon. Caused by atmospheric scattering.

magnetic compass   A compass using the earth's magnetic field as the directional force.

magnetic dip   A freely suspended magnetised needle will not only line up horizontally in the earth's field, but will lie at an angle with the horizon. This angle between the needle and the plane of the horizon is called magnetic dip.

magnetic equator   A line joining places with zero dip. A freely suspended needle would hang horizontal to the earth's surface. At the magnetic poles, where the needle would point directly downward, the dip is 90°.

magnetic north   The direction of the magnetic north pole from any point on the surface of the earth.

Maritime air   Air which has blown a long distance over the sea and is therefore moist.

mark   A fixed feature on the land or moored at sea, which can be identified on the chart and used to fix the boat's position.

mean sea level (MSL)   The mean level of the sea computed by measurement of the hourly heights of tide during complete tidal cycles for periods of a month or of a year, and averaging the results.

Mercator chart   A chart drawn on the Mercator projection. Rhumb lines can be drawn as straight lines but great circles appear as curves.

meridian A great circle passing through the earth's true poles which, in practical terms, gives a north-south reference line.

millibar (mb) see hectopascal.

navigation Navigation is the art of taking a vessel in safety from one place to another, as economically as possible.

navigation lights Lights on a craft to give warning of its presence, aspect and occupation.

overfalls or tide rips Turbulence caused when strong tidal streams flow over abrupt changes in depth, or with the meeting of tidal streams flowing from different directions.

pay off A boat pays off if her bow falls away from the wind.

pitch/pitching Rotation about the beam axis of a boat – In practice the rising and falling of the bow and stern due to the action of the waves or swells.

pitchpoling Capsizing by somersaulting over the bow. A boat moving too fast down the face of a wave may push her bow into the rear of the wave ahead, and pitchpole over her bow onto her deck.

plan position indicator (PPI) A radar display showing, as on a chart, the positions of other echo-producing vessels or marks and the outline of the coast.

plot Diagrammatic representation of the progress of a craft, usually on a chart.

Polar Maritime airstream Air blowing from the antarctic region which is cool and moist.

port To the left, looking forward in a boat. Denoted by the colour red.

position line or line of position (LOP) A line on a chart on which the boat lies or has lain. It may be straight, curved, or irregular in shape.

pounding Continual forcible impact between hull and waves when the forepart of a pitching vessel lifts out of the water and the full weight slams bodily down into the next wave trough.

projection The representation on the plane surface of a chart of all or any part of the curved surface of the earth.

pushpit A tubing structure in the stern of the boat, similar to the bow pulpit.

Racon A radar beacon which responds to a craft's radar transmissions by transmitting a signal that appears as a radial line on the PPI.

radar Use of reflected radio waves to find distance and/or bearing of objects. Initial letters of Radio Aid to Detection And Ranging.

radar relative display A PPI on which the user's boat remains stationary (generally in the centre).

radio direction finding (RDF) Finding the bearing of a radio transmitting aerial by means of a loop or other directional receiving aerial.

Ramark   A radar beacon that transmits independently of any triggering pulse from ships' radars. The signal appears as a broken radial line on the PPI.

range (of light)   In general, the distance at which a light can be seen. In particular, geographical range: maximum theoretical distance at which a light can be seen limited only by height of eye of the observer, height of the light, curvature of the earth and normal atmospheric refraction. Luminous range: theoretical distance a light may be sighted depending on the intensity (brightness) of the light, and irrespective of its elevation or observer's height of eye. Nominal range: distance a light can be seen when the actual visibility is 10 miles. Used in light descriptions on charts converted to metric units.

range (radar)   The distance of an object detected on radar, measured on the radar display.

relative (direction)   Direction in the horizontal plane with reference to the bow of a boat. An object dead ahead is 0°REL. Measured clockwise through 360°, or through 180° to port or starboard when it may be prefixed red or green.

repeater   A device for repeating at a distance the indications of an instrument such as a compass, where the readings of the master compass would be available at various positions in a boat.

rhumb line   A line that cuts all meridians at the same angle: line followed by a craft sailing on one course.

roll/rolling   Rotation about the longitudinal axis of a boat. In particular the alternate inclination of a craft from side to side away from the upright position due to the action of the waves, especially when on the beam. Can cause extreme nausea.

running fix   A fix in which position lines are not obtained simultaneously but the first is run or transferred to the time of the second.

Secondary port   A port for which tidal data is given in national Tidal Tables, but for which daily predictions are not given.

scud   To drive before a gale either under bare poles, or with only enough sail to steady the craft. Also low, broken clouds that fly swiftly before the wind.

sea   The name given to waves generated by wind blowing locally.

set (of current)   The direction of movement of a current or tidal stream.

set and drift   The difference bewteen a DR position on the chart — but *not* an EP — and a fix for the same time is termed set and drift. The direction from the DR to the fix, which can be measured on the compass rose, is termed set, and the distance in nautical miles is termed drift.

small circle   Any circle on the surface of the earth other than a great circle, e.g., all parallels of latitude, other than the equator, are small circles.

Southern Alps   Chain of mountains, including seventeen peaks over

3,000 metres, running entire length of south island of New Zealand.

Standard port A port for which daily predictions of high and low water are given in national Tide Tables.

starboard To the right, looking forward in a boat. Denoted by the colour green.

swell Waves which have been generated at a distance, usually by a storm, or the residual waves in an area when the wind has ceased to blow.

topmark A special shape secured at the top of a buoy or beacon to aid identification.

track The future or intended path of a vessel.

Traffic Separation Scheme A scheme which aims at reducing the risk of collision in areas which are either congested or converging, or both, by separating traffic moving in opposite, or nearly opposite directions into traffic lanes.

trim The inclination of a boat in the fore-and-aft sense (pitch). A boat with no trim is floating on 'an even keel'. To trim 'by the head' or 'by the stern' is to have a bow down or bow up attitude.

Tropical Maritime airstream Air blowing from the tropics which is warm and moist.

trough The hollow between two successive waves.

true direction Direction measured clockwise from true north through 360°.

true motion display A PPI that compensates for the course and speed of the user's craft so that fixed objects such as navigation buoys or land remain stationary on the radar display.

true north The direction from any point on the earth to the true north pole.

variation (magnetic) The angle at a place between the direction of true north and the direction of magnetic north. Named east if magnetic north lies to the right of true north, otherwise, west.

veer The wind is said to veer when it changes direction clockwise or to the right, e.g., from north to north-east, or south to south-west.

vertical The direction of gravity.

wave An undulation of the sea surface. The water particles rise and fall and may achieve a rotary motion as the wave passes, but do not move horizontally with the wave.

water track Actual direction or true course made good through the water after applying leeway to course steered. In still water it is the same as ground track. Where there is also a crosstide or current, the water track stays the same, but the ground track changes.

wave train A group or series of related waves.

weatherfax A weather facsimile receiver which gives an instant printout of a weather map, showing highs, lows, fronts and isobars.

wind shear A change in wind speed in a short distance at right angles across the direction of the wind. Commonly used to describe the change of wind speed with height which is vertical (wind) shear, but it can also act in a horizontal direction and, occasionally, in both. The degree of turbulence increases as the amount of wind shear increases.

yaw Unavoidable oscillation of the boat's head either side of the course being steered or when at anchor, due to wind and waves.

Index

Units, chart symbols for 16
    depth 15
    distance at sea 6
    of force 177
    pressure 128, 177
    speed at sea 6
    wind speed 125

valley wind 127, 177
variation, magnetic 49, 51
variables (winds) 131
veer 181
vertical danger angle 118
  sextant angle (VSA) 115
    taking 117
visibility of lights 34, 36, 89–90

warm fronts 137–8
water track 74, 181
wave train 148
waves 139–40, 146, 181

weather 128–53
    facsimile receiver 181
    forecasting 140–1
    lore 142
    map 141
westerlies 124
wind 119–30
    Beaufort, scale of 122–3
    causes of 120
    direction 120, 133, 145
    fohn 136, 176
    katabatic 127, 177
    shear 134, 181
    speed 125
      diurnal variation in 136
winds 120–5
    local 125
    trade 124
    valley (katabatic) 127, 177
    variables 124